PHYSIOLOGY AND PATHOLOGY
IN THE PERINATAL PERIOD

BOERHAAVE SERIES FOR POSTGRADUATE MEDICAL EDUCATION

PROCEEDINGS OF THE BOERHAAVE COURSES
ORGANIZED BY
THE FACULTY OF MEDICINE, UNIVERSITY OF LEIDEN,
THE NETHERLANDS

PHYSIOLOGY AND PATHOLOGY IN THE PERINATAL PERIOD

EDITED BY

R. H. GEVERS, M.D. AND J. H. RUYS, M.D.

Leiden University Hospital

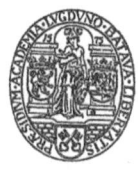

LEIDEN UNIVERSITY PRESS

1971

SOLE DISTRIBUTOR FOR NORTH AMERICA
SPRINGER-VERLAG NEW YORK INC. / NEW YORK

ISBN-13: 978-94-010-3150-9   e-ISBN-13978-94-010-3148-6
DOI: 10.1007/978-94-010-3148-6

Library of Congress Catalog Card Number 76–140618

Jacket design: E. Wijnans

CONTENTS

LIST OF CONTRIBUTORS

G. S. Dawes, The Nuffield Institute for Medical Research, University of Oxford, U.K.

T. K. A. B. Eskes, Department of Obstetrics, St. Lucas Hospital, Amsterdam, Netherlands

J. Favier, Department of Obstetrics and Gynecology, University Hospital, Leiden, Netherlands

J. L. J. Gaillard, Pathological Laboratory, University of Leiden, Netherlands

H. H. van Gelderen, Department of Pediatrics, University Hospital, Leiden, Netherlands

R. H. Gevers, Department of Obstetrics and Gynecology, University Hospital, Leiden, Netherlands

F. Kubli, Department of Obstetrics, University Hospital, Basel, Switzerland

D. H. G. Keuskamp, Department of Anesthesiology, Dijkzigt University Hospital, Rotterdam, Netherlands

R. de Leeuw, Department of Physiology and Pathology of the Newborn, Wilhelmina Hospital, University of Amsterdam, Netherlands

D. T. Popescu, Department of Anesthesiology, University Hospital, Leiden, Netherlands

P. E. R. Rhemrev, Department of Obstetrics and Gynecology, University Hospital, Leiden, Netherlands

H. Rüttgers, Department of Obstetrics, University Hospital, Basel, Switzerland

J. H. Ruys, Neonatal Unit, Department of Obstetrics and gynecology, University Hospital, Leiden, Netherlands

H. J. Shelley, The Nuffield Institute for Medical Research, University of Oxford, U.K.

A. Sikkel, Department of Obstetrics and Gynecology, University Hospital, Leiden, Netherlands

J. Spierdijk, Department of Anesthesiology, University Hospital, Leiden, Netherlands

J. J. van Zanten, Intensive Care Unit, University Hospital, Leiden, Netherlands

PARTICIPANTS IN THE DISCUSSION *

J. van Aken, Anesthesist, Drongen, Belgium
J. W. Barents, Obstetrician and gynecologist, Arnhem
J. H. van Bemmel, Institute of Medical Physics T.N.O., University of Utrecht
M. A. Broer, Pediatrician, Assen
J. I. de Bruijne, Department of Physiology and Pathology of the Newborn, Wilhelmina Gasthuis, University of Amsterdam
A. C. Drogendijk, Department of Obstetrics and Gynecology, Free University, Amsterdam
H. D. Hamming, Pediatrician, Groningen
J. J. van der Harten, Pathological anatomist, Amstelveen
M. J. Koop, Pediatrician, Brunsum
J. G. Koppe, Pediatrician, Amsterdam
J. Lauweryns, Department of Pathological Anatomy, University Hospital Saint Raphaël, Louvain, Belgium
H. A. Polman, Pediatrician, Haren (Gr.)
J. Reepmaker, Pediatrician, Dordrecht
R. L. Rosan, Stanford University, U.S.A.
A. A. M. de Steenhuijsen Piters, Pediatrician, Oosterhout (N.-B.)
J. G. Stolk, Gynecologist, Arnhem

* When country is not indicated, address in the Netherlands.

PREFACE

The course of history is never one of smooth progression. Periods of relative quietness are interrupted by periods of wars and revolution. This pattern resembles that of a river which, before flowing into the delta, has to pass countless rapids. The same holds for the development of the science of medicine. In obstetrics some of these 'revolutions' or 'rapids' consist of the introduction of conservative obstetrical treatment by Lucas Johann Boer at the beginning of the nineteenth century, the discovery of the cause of puerperal sepsis by Oliver Wendell Holmes and Semmelweiss between 1843 and 1847, the introduction of the principle of asepsis by Pasteur in 1874, the introduction of prenatal care at the end of the nineteenth and the beginning of the twentieth century (Mijnlieff, Treub, De Snoo), the improvement of surgical techniques, the possibility to treat shock by bloodtransfusion, and, finally, the acquisition of new means for the effective therapy of infection. All these developments have led to a sharp reduction of maternal and perinatal mortality.

In this connection it must be pointed out that such a reduction could never have been accomplished without the favourable social changes as a result of which medical and prenatal care could be made universally available. In recent years there has been another revolutionary development in obstetrics. Two factors have been responsible for this: the application of basic sciences in obstetrics, and the dissolution of the isolation with respect to other clinical disciplines. Our knowledge and views have been increased since the physiological processes during pregnancy and labour have been studied in collaboration with physiologists and biochemists. For indeed, how can we know where pathology starts if we are ignorant of the physiology? Between these two regions lies a 'no-man's-land', whose area is now steadily diminishing.

Modern obstetrics must concentrate on perinatal morbidity. The immense difficulties involved in this subject can be judged from the fact that we have not yet been able to define, even in adults, just what illness is.

There is no doubt that the historia morbi is of great importance for arriving at the correct diagnosis in a patient and that the historia morbi of the newborn belongs mainly to the period of intra-uterine life. Until recently, we obstetricians had a far too simple conception of this exceedingly important period in human life. For us too, it holds that 'l'interpretation simpliste des causes a toujours faussé l'histoire' (Gustave le Bon).

It is clear to all of us that the responsibility accepted by every scientist, namely the search for truth, cannot be the responsibility of the obstetrician alone. Close collaboration with physiologists, biochemists, paediatricians, anaesthesists and pathologists is imperative.

This is the view that has governed the composition of the present program, both the subjects and the speakers. We are happy that so many of you were able to accept our invitation to participate, whether as speakers or as listeners.

Today we are mainly concerned with 'the intra-uterine patient'. As Le Bon put it: 'Dans la genèse des phenomènes historiques les causes s'additionnent en progression arithmétique et leurs effects en progression géométrique', and this certainly does not differ for the treatment of perinatal pathology. The smallest disturbances occurring during intra-uterine life can at a given moment have great and serious consequences. This is why it is of paramount importance to detect the possible causes of perinatal *morbidity* as early and as thoroughly as possible, which will give therapy its greatest chance of success.

A. SIKKEL M.D.
University Hospital, Leiden

GAS EXCHANGE BETWEEN MOTHER AND
FOETUS AND PLACENTAL DESIGN

G. S. DAWES

Our knowledge of placental gas exchange and of foetal blood gas homeostasis is based largely upon animal models and abstract calculations.
There has been a revolution in our understanding of these problems in the
last few years, as a result of the introduction of new techniques and the
greater number of investigators. So this is an appropriate time at which
to survey the scene.

Placental gas exchange depends on many factors. Some of these have
been extensively studied and are very well known. They include the special
characteristics of maternal and foetal blood (the size of the O_2 carrying
capacity and the shape and position of the Hb-O_2 and CO_2 dissociation
curves). We recognize that a proper understanding of these are a necessary
prerequisite to physiological studies on placental gas exchange. Yet so
much has been written about them that one might be forgiven for supposing that they constituted the single most important variable. From the
practical point of view, however, they are factors which are not readily
accessible to manipulation in vivo. They can be altered only by intrauterine transfusion or, perhaps, by changes in the erythropoietin concentration of the blood. Replacement of foetal with maternal blood in lambs at
0.67–0.86 of term (with a large shift to the right in the Hb-O_2 dissociation
curve) caused a fall in umbilical vein O_2 saturation and a rise in PO_2 but
no systematic changes of blood flows or O_2 consumption rates (1). Human
foetuses also survive both thorough transfusion *in utero* and (in erythroblastosis foetalis) a very low O_2 capacity of the circulating blood.

Another factor about which much has been written, but of which we
know little for certain, is the geometry of the flow pathways in the area of
gas exchange. There are four possible arrangements, countercurrent flow,
concurrent, crosscurrent (or multivillous) and 'pool' flow systems. It is
probable that in the placenta of some species more than one such flow
pathway may coexist. For instance in the only situation which has been

subjected to experimental analysis, the placenta of the sheep, Metcalfe, Bartels, Hilpert and Parer (2), using the inert gases N_2O and CO and reversing the direction of umbilical flow, concluded that it was a mixture of concurrent and countercurrent flow systems. The countercurrent system would be the most efficient for gaseous exchange, but the placenta is certainly not designed that way.

We also distinguish between those placentas which have defined vascular channels on both the foetal and maternal sides (as in the sheep) and those in which the maternal channels within the intervillous space are less well defined (as in primates). We still have no satisfactory experimental evidence as to the size or geometry of the maternal flow pathways in haemochorial primate placentas. It may be a crosscurrent system (often described as multivillous) but it is important at this time to recognize that we do not know.

MATERNAL PLACENTAL BLOOD FLOW

We now turn to a consideration of a variable which should to some extent be under control, in the experimental laboratory if not in the clinic, that is, maternal placental blood flow. However, this is far from being the case. Although uterine arterial or venous blood flows have been measured by direct methods (by attachment of uterine arterial flow probes or collection of venous effluent) or by indirect methods (by an application of the Fick principle using either nitrous oxide or 4-aminoantipyrine) for many years, these do not give a measure of maternal *placental* blood flow. The proportion of uterine flow to the maternal side of the placenta, to the myometrium, endometrium, cervix, vagina, tubes and adnexae has been uncertain. It is only within the last year and for the first time that the distribution of uterine blood flow has been measured. The method used has been injection of isotope-labelled microspheres (3, 4). The principle of the method is that the isotope-labelled microspheres are injected into the systemic circulation so that they are well mixed (usually by a left intraventricular injection); they are of a size ($25–50\mu$) such that they impact in the smaller arterioles. Only a small proportion, normally less than 2%, are found in the lungs and of these most have arrived via the bronchial arteries. Shortly before the microspheres are injected a pump is started which withdraws blood steadily at a known rate (e.g. 5 ml/min.) from an artery; the pump is stopped about 15 secs after the end of the injection, by which time all the microspheres are impacted, some of them in the withdrawal syringe. If at postmortem the radioactivity in a kidney is 10 times that in the withdrawal syringe then the renal blood flow must have been 50 ml per minute at the time of the injection. By using several different isotopes, whose activity can be measured in the presence of others, it is possible to make several independent measurements of flow. The flow to any organ or tissue that can be anatomically separated, and thus counted separately, can be distinguished.

Using this method in the pregnant rabbit near term Duncan and Lewis (3) found that hypoxaemia caused a large fall in maternal placental blood flow, while myometrial flow was unaltered. In her most recent paper Duncan (4) found that reducing the maternal arterial PO_2 from 86 to 35 mmHg (with little change in PCO_2) caused a fall in maternal placental blood flow from 20.0 ± 1.4 to 13.1 ± 2.2 ml/min., whereas myometrial flow was 6.7 ± 0.8 ml/min. while breathing air and 7.8 ± 1.2 ml/min. while breathing an hypoxic gas micture. So in this experimental situation the proportion of uterine flow which was distributed to the maternal side of the placenta altered very considerably. Consequently in the future we can place no reliance on measurements of total uterine flow as a measure of what may be reaching the placenta, other than as an upper limit.

Now that we have an experimental tool which enables us to measure maternal placental flow it should be possible to study the physiological control mechanisms. The decrease in maternal placental blood flow observed during maternal hypoxaemia in the rabbit might be due to liberation of catecholamines into the circulating bloodstream or by liberation of other vasoactive substances or by direct sympathetic or parasympathetic neural control. It remains to be seen whether the same method can be applied satisfactorily to the primate placenta. Rabbits are cheap and lend themselves comparatively well as an experimental model for studying the problems, but they are notoriously susceptible to changes in their environment, and often produce runts or dead foetuses in their relatively large litters. Nevertheless small-for-dates infants are known in man, and such studies may give us an insight into the mechanisms which may be at work in the primate placenta, which is so much more difficult to study.

The same general mechanism may be at work in different species. In pregnant guinea pigs (5) and sheep (6) maternal hypocapnia sufficient to reduce the maternal PCO_2 below 20 mmHg was associated with a deterioration in the term foetus, shown by a fall in umbilical venous or arterial PO_2 or, in the extreme case, progressive metabolic acidosis. We have seen the same phenomenon in pregnant sheep though in our hands the effect has not been so severe as hitherto reported; maternal hypocapnia (PCO_2

< 20 mmHg) was associated with a fall in foetal carotid PO_2 of 3–4 mmHg. The explanations offered by previous workers have been various and have included changes both in the mother and in the foetus. The most likely explanation, and that most widely canvassed, is that maternal hypocapnia is associated with a decrease in maternal placental blood flow. In unpublished observations Dr. B. Le Duc has found that maternal hypocapnia in rabbits near term is associated with a fall in maternal placental flow of a size which, were it to occur in other species, could have explained the deterioration in the condition of the foetus. As with hypoxaemia so with hypocapnia the question arises as to what mechanism is involved, direct or indirect. Until we know the answers to these questions it may be wise to avoid both hypoxaemia and hypocapnia, and to recognize that we still have a lot to learn about the fundamental mechanism which may be involved.

Finally these observations should make us even more cautious than hitherto about the use of indirect methods for measuring maternal placental bloodflow. It is evident that methods which give an estimate of the clearance of radioactive material from the myometrium or which rely on the interpretation of changes in temperature in uterine or cervical muscle might well give a very misleading impression of what is happening within the placenta itself.

It is also interesting to note that, in the only two species examined (sheep (7); dog, (8) blood samples from maternal placental venules had a PO_2 which was variable (suggesting placental inhomogeneity, defined below) and widely different from that in myometrial or uterine venous blood. The latter, therefore, is a poor index of placental venous effluent.

PLACENTAL METABOLISM

The placenta is a vigorous metabolic organ which consumes oxygen and produces CO_2. In sheep this metabolism takes place within or in series with the area of gas exchange (7). The evidence for this was obtained by replacing the foetal lamb by a warmed reservoir and pump filled with foetal blood; the placenta remained intact *in utero* and the pump circulated blood through the foetal side of the placenta via the umbilical vessels. The pump neither consumed nor released oxygen or CO_2 and within a few minutes from starting it the blood flowing through the foetal side of the placenta came into equilibrium, so that the gas contents and tensions of the umbilical arterial and venous bloods were identical. In these circumstances the PO_2 of the blood in the umbilical vessels on the foetal side of the placenta was about 40–45 mm Hg below the normal arterial PO_2 on the maternal side of the placenta (about 90 mm Hg). Thus the transplacental gradient for O_2, due to oxygen consumption within the placenta alone, and in the absence of the foetus, was 40–45 mm Hg; the gradient for PCO_2 is about 7 mm Hg (unpublished). The total gradient between maternal arterial and foetal carotid arterial blood for oxygen is about 70 mm Hg and for CO_2 about 14 mm Hg. So we can say that approximately half the transplacental gas tension gradient is due to placental metabolism and about half is due to a combination of placental inhomogeneity, foetal metabolism and the geometry of the foetal circulation. This observation explains, incidentally, why it is so difficult to induce large changes in foetal PO_2 by administering high oxygen mixtures to the mother. It is also evident that the placenta is in a preemptive position compared with the foetus in respect of gas exchange; that is to say it has priority over the foetus. In the anaesthetized pregnant sheep near term the oxygen uptake of the placenta was rather more than a third of that of the foetus. Perhaps placental metabolism also affects the transplacental gradient for substances other than the blood gases.

UMBILICAL BLOOD FLOW

Experiments on foetal lambs by many observers have shown that umbilical blood flow is a large proportion of total cardiac output, about 50%, and does not vary much with age over the last half of gestation. Flow is of the order of 200 ml/kg foetal body weight per minute. Such measurements as have been made on man are consistent with a figure of this size, taking into account the greater difficulty in making such measurements after delivery. To get this figure in perspective one has to remember that in large animals, including man, basal cardiac output is 70–80 ml/kg min.

In vivo over a wide physiological range of blood gas values, umbilical vascular resistance did not vary significantly, even when foetal arterial PO_2 was greatly increased on ventilation. The umbilical vessels also seemed relatively insensitive to catecholamines. To produce vasoconstriction it was necessary to infuse intravenously doses of 1 μg/kg min noradrenaline or more. So it was concluded that umbilical vascular resistance (through the foetal side of the placenta) was low and relatively invariable under normal physiological circumstances (9). Now it is recognized that this opinion runs contrary to that often expressed by workers who have used the isolated perfused cords or placentas obtained after human delivery. Such preparations have been described as highly susceptible to changes in the PO_2 of the perfusion fluid. The discrepancy is more apparent than real. It is difficult to obtain in an isolated perfused preparation, even one from a recently delivered sheep foetus, conditions which approximate to those observed in vivo with the umbilical circulation intact. The umbilical cord vessels of the sheep, perfused in vitro, react in much the same way as those obtained from human material (10). Yet in vivo it is possible to alter foetal arterial PO_2 from 15–65 mm Hg with no discernable change in umbilical vascular resistance.

Hence the general picture emerges that umbilical vascular resistance is relatively low and relatively invariant, conditions which are rational for an organ of gaseous exchange. This does not mean that umbilical blood flow does not alter. It can be altered considerably by relatively small changes in arterial blood pressure, as shown below.

PLACENTAL HOMOGENEITY

If the placenta were functionally homogeneous from a vascular point of view, (i.e. the ratio maternal placental: umbilical flow were equal in every unit of the gas exchanging area) the efficiency of gas exchange would be greater than if it were inhomogeneous. An extreme instance of inhomogeneity of flow is illustrated by a situation in which part of the placenta on the maternal side, e.g. the 'supporting structure', is supplied by maternal blood but not by foetal blood; this constitutes a shunt on the maternal side. Similarly foetal blood may supply part of the foetal side of the placenta, e.g. the supporting structures of the villous trees, which do not receive maternal blood, and hence constitute a shunt on the foetal side. Aherne and Dunnill (11) calculated that such supporting structures constituted about a fifth of the human placenta. This type of inhomogeneity has been described as variations in the perfusion: perfusion ratio (12) by analogy with variations in the ventilation: perfusion ratio of the lung. There are two other sources of inhomogeneity; first, variations in placental permeability and, secondly, variations in metabolic rate in different placental units. Two questions arise. First is it possible to estimate the degree of inhomogeneity, and secondly can we speculate as to what physiological factors may influence it?

The only attempt so far to measure the perfusion: perfusion ratio in the placenta of sheep (13) used macroaggregated albumen particles labelled with ^{125}I or ^{131}I injected on either side of the placenta. There are obvious difficulties in the interpretation of these results related to the fact that gas exchange takes place between capillaries rather than between the arterioles in which the particles were impacted and also to the fact that the distribution of such particulate matter on either side of the placenta is random. However this is an interesting attempt to solve a problem of great technical difficulty; debate on the interpretation is bound to continue. On the second question, that of physiological control, we as yet know nothing, though it is worthwhile considering briefly the situation in the lung. In the lung ventilation with an hypoxic gas mixture leads to vasoconstriction, and this has been interpreted as a mechanism by which the ventilation: perfusion ratio might be adjusted within individual units of the lung. Conversely in the placenta it is conceivable that perfusion with, for instance, a relatively hypoxic foetal blood might lead to vasodilatation on the maternal side or vice versa. It is easier to see how this might happen in the placenta of the sheep or rabbit rather than in the haemochorial placenta of the primate. So far as I am aware noone has tackled this problem experimentally, though it is now just coming within the range of experimental possibility.

If a large part of the transplacental gradient for the respiratory gases is due to placental metabolism, and if a further part can be attributed to placental inhomogeneity, it must follow that the placental barrier to gaseous diffusion is much less than hitherto supposed. This is so. Longo et al. (13, 14) found the diffusion capacity for CO and O_2 to be relatively high, with an estimated mean maternal – foetal PO_2 gradient of only 6.3 mm Hg in sheep near term. This compares favourably with Barron and Meschia's (15) original estimate of 33–48 mm Hg.

FOETAL BLOOD GAS HOMEOSTASIS

After birth, and given a reasonably efficient lung and circulation, blood gas homeostasis depends on the chemoreceptors, the central chemoreceptors in the floor of the fourth ventricle and the systemic arterial chemoreceptors in the carotid and aortic bodies. They control the circulation and the breathing. However in foetal life the lungs are not yet expanded and breathing movements are said to be uncommon; the placenta rather than the lungs is the organ of gaseous exchange. So far as we yet know neither the central nor the carotid chemoreceptors are functionally active in the foetus, so the foetal circulation is largely controlled by the aortic chemoreceptors (and of course the arterial baroreceptors). The principal evidence for this is that moderate degrees of hypoxaemia in foetal lambs over the range PO_2 40–15 mm Hg causes a progressive rise of arterial pressure and hindlimb vasoconstriction. These phenomena are abolished by section of the aortic nerves or of the cervical vagi which they join (16). Denervation of the carotid bifurcations does not affect the response. Moderate hypoxaemia excites the aortic chemoreceptors to cause tachycardia, a rise of foetal arterial pressure and a redistribution of cardiac output with an increase in umbilical blood flow. The aortic bodies exert a tonic effect upon the foetal circulation as shown by the fact that section of the aortic nerves or of the cervical vagi causes a fall of arterial pressure, an increase in the hindlimb blood flow and much reduces the ability of the foetus to withstand short episodes of hypoxia or asphyxia.

In the foetal lamb this aortic body control of the circulation comes into play during the latter half of gestation. It has long been known that in the adult excitation of the aortic bodies has a large effect upon the circulation and a comparatively small effect upon breathing. This seems admirably suited for the predimment role of the aortic chemoreceptors in foetal life. It is also interesting to note that the first effects of mild hypoxaemia on the human foetus is to cause tachycardia, and it is tempting to suppose that this is due to stimulation primarily of the aortic chemoreceptors. The sensitivity of this system to hypoxaemia is also dependent on the level of the arterial PCO_2, that is to say a given degree of hypoxaemia in the foetal lamb has a greater effect during hypercapnia.

FOETAL ACTIVITY IN ANAESTHESIA

Changes in foetal activity certainly occur, and greater muscular activity must temporarily increase oxygen requirements. We must also consider the possibility that the foetus has periods of quiescence approximating to sleep, in which its respiratory gas exchange will be considerably less. The course of the foetal circulation is such that an increase in foetal oxygen consumption will lead inevitably to a small fall in foetal carotid PO_2 and vice versa. This is a complication to the interpretation of human foetal scalp sampling which is often overlooked. It partly explains why pH rather than PO_2 levels are a more useful indication of foetal wellbeing.

We may also briefly consider the effect of general anaesthesia. If general anaesthesia is sufficient to abolish muscular tone this of itself will reduce oxygen consumption. The normal oxygen consumption of unanaesthetised newborn rhesus monkeys in a neutral thermal environment at rest or sleeping is about 9.5 ml/kg min; under light pentobarbitone anaesthesia it is about 7.5 ml/kg min. Qualitatively similar results have been observed in newborn rabbits and guinea pigs. Barbiturate anaesthesia has some other interesting effects which are worth a brief mention. Thus in rhesus monkeys near term the brains of newly delivered infants were removed for histo-pathological examination, after the infants were asphyxiated for 12½ minutes, and were then resuscitated and allowed to live some weeks or months. As compared with delivery under local anaesthesia, administration of barbiturate to the mother, to provide light general anaesthesia for a period of 30 minutes before delivery, had the effect of substantially increasing the ease of resuscitation of the infant and greatly reduced or, in some instances, wholly prevented permanent brain damage. It should perhaps be emphasized that these experiments were done not as a model for man but to test the effects of barbiturate anaesthesia in a controlled experimental situation. I would not yet advocate the extension of the results to clinical practice. For one thing, we cannot be sure that pentobarbitone (the barbiturate actually used) is the most satisfactory agent, and it can have some disadvantages in practice. This is a subject which may deserve further exploration.

CONCLUSION

The physiology of transplacental gas exchange and, what is equally important, the physiology of foetal reactions to changes in its blood gases, form a complex, fascinating and closely integrated system. In this paper I have tried to emphasize the biological variables which might be of greater interest to the obstetrician as being more or less susceptible of control. Thus we may hope to be able to exercise some control, not only on maternal blood gases, but (perhaps by means of drugs) on maternal placental blood flow and indirectly upon the foetus. We are aware that the foetus plays a very active part, so that drugs which affect the autonomic nervous system of the mother can also affect that of the foetus. It is obvious that care will have to be exercised to use such drugs intelligently; there is little virtue in using an agent which improves the circulation to the maternal side of the placenta if it disturbs physiological control of the foetal circulation.

I began by saying that we have seen a revolution in our attitude to placental physiology. It used to be thought that the placenta was designed so as to facilitate gas transfer. We know now that the vascular architecture is not the most efficient, that metabolism takes place in the area of gas exchange, and there are reasons, histological and experimental, for supposing that there is a degree of placental inhomogeneity which introduces a further element of inefficiency. On the other hand the so-called diffusion barrier seems to have been lowered to an extent where it has little practical influence on physiological transfer.

Evidently the basic design of the placenta is predicated on considerations other than gas exchange. There are immunological and hormonal considerations. The normal placenta appears to provide an effective barrier to cellular transfer between mother and foetus, and is probably an essential (though not the only) factor in protecting the foetus against the immunological hazard from its mother (17). The placenta provides a supply of hormones, chorionic gonadotrophin, steroid and lactogen, some of which are essential for the maintenance of pregnancy. And finally it is designed for rapid growth and disposal, from a phylogenetic constitution of remote antiquity. It is hardly surprising that its gas exchanging function should be of secondary importance in design, though its importance to foetal survival is vital.

REFERENCES

1. Meschia G., Battaglia F. C., Makowski E. L. and Droegemueller W. *J. appl. Physiol.* 26, 410–415 (1969).
2. Metcalfe J., Moll W., Bartels H., Hilpert P. and Parer J. T., *Circulation Res.* 16, 95–101 (1965).
3. Duncan S. L. B. and Lewis B. V., *J. Physiol.* 202, 471–481 (1969)
4. Duncan S. L. B., *J. Physiol.* 204, 421–434 (1969).
5. Morishima H. O., Daniel S. S., Adamsons K. and James L. S., *Amer. J. Obst. Gynec.* 93, 269–273 (1965).
6. Motoyama E. K., Rivard G., Acheson F. and Cook C. D., *Lancet* 1, 286–288 (1966).
7. Campbell A. G. M., Dawes G. S., Fishman A. P., Hyman A. I. and James G. B. *J. Physiol.* 182, 439–464 (1966).
8. Longo L. D., Schwarz R. H. and Forster R. E., *J. appl. Physiol.*, 24 787–791 (1968).
9. Dawes G. S., *Foetal and Neonatal Physiology.* Year Book Medical Publishers, Chicago (1968).
10. Lewis B. V., *J. Obstet. Gynec. Brit. Cwlth.* 75, 87–91 (1968).
11. Aherne W. and Dunnill M. S., *J. Path. Bact.* 91, 123–140 (1966).
12. Dawes G. S., *Handbook of Physiology, Respiration II* 1313–1328 (1965).
13. Longo L. D., Power G. G. and Forster R. E., *J. Clin. Invest.* 46, 812–828 (1967).
14. Longo L. D., Power G. G. and Forster R. E., *J. appl. Physiol.* 26, 360–370 (1969).
15. Barron D. H. and Meschia G., *Cold. Spring Harb. Symp. Quant. Biol.* 19, 93–101 (1954).
16. Dawes G. S., Duncan S. L. B., Lewis B. V., Merlet C. L., Owen-Thomas J. B. and Reeves J. T., *J. Physiol.* 201, 117–128 (1969).
17. Billington W. D., Kirby D. R. S., Owen J. J. T., Ritter M. A., Burtonshaw M. D., Evans E. P., Ford C. E., Gauld I. K. and McLaren A. *Nature* 224, 704–706 (1969).

GLUCOSE METABOLISM IN THE FOETUS IN PHYSIOLOGICAL AND PATHOLOGICAL CIRCUMSTANCES

H. J. SHELLEY

THE ROLE OF GLUCOSE IN THE NORMAL FOETUS

Glucose of maternal origin is thought to be both the principal substrate for oxidative metabolism in the foetus and the main precursor for the synthesis of foetal glycogen, triglycerides and other lipids. This belief is derived from attempts to study *a*) the permeability of the placenta to various substances, *b*) their rate of uptake by the foetus, and *c*) the ability of foetal tissues to utilize them as a source of energy or for synthetic purposes. Figure 1 attempts to summarize the rather small body of information available and is a generalized scheme, taking no account of possible species differences.

Glocose has been shown to cross the placenta readily in several species, including man, and is thought to do so by 'facilitated diffusion'; i.e. it passes across the placenta in the direction of the diffusion gradient, but at a faster rate than can be explained by simple diffusion (1). Since the

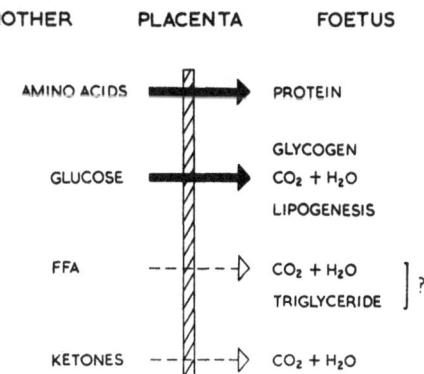

Fig. 1. A diagram to illustrate the permeability of the placenta to substances of maternal origin and their fate in the foetus.

maternal blood glucose concentration is usually higher than that in the foetus (see below), glucose normally passes from mother to foetus. The glucose concentration in the umbilical vein is normally higher than that in the umbilical artery and in human babies at delivery calculation from the mean umbilical arterio-venous difference for glucose, 8–12 mg/100 ml (2, 3, 4, 5, 6), and the mean umbilical blood flow, 75 ml/kg/min. (7), suggests that the foetal glucose uptake is about 8 mg/kg/min. If all the glucose were oxidized, this would correspond to an oxygen consumption of 6.5 ml/kg/min. Since all actual oxygen consumption of the foetus in utero probably approximates to the minimal oxygen consumption of the newborn baby, 4.8 ml/kg/min. (8), the calculated glucose uptake is sufficient both to maintain oxidative metabolism and provide glucose for synthetic purposes. A few observations on foetal lambs suggest that in this species also the uptake of glucose may be sufficient to support oxidative metabolism (9, 10).

This conclusion is supported by studies of the placental transfer and foetal uptake of other substances. Amino acids must cross the placenta in amounts sufficient to support foetal growth, and they appear to do so against the concentration gradient (1), but in vitro studies suggest that in the dog and rat the ability of the liver to degrade amino acids does not develop until after birth (11, 12, 13); presumably they are conserved for protein synthesis. Studies on the sheep, rabbit and rat suggest that the placenta is only slightly permeable to free fatty acids (14, 15, 16, 34). The low foetal plasma level and small umbilical arterio-venous difference for free fatty acids in man, first observed by van Duyne and Havel (1959), has been confirmed repeatedly and suggests that the foetal uptake of free fatty acids is probably less than 1 mg/kg min even at high maternal plasma concentrations. Since studies on the foetal rabbit and sheep suggest that little or no fatty acid is oxidized by the foetus (17, 18), it is likely that any taken up by the foetus is retained in the foetal lipids. The foetal lamb is able to utilize acetate and oxidize ketone bodies, but the placental permeability to these substances is low and the foetus does not synthesize ketones (20, 21, 22). In man, some placental transfer and foetal uptake of ketones does occur when the mother has a high blood ketone level (23, 24). No net foetal uptake of glycerol occurs in either sheep or man (25, 24).

During the latter part of gestation both lipid and glycogen accumulate in the foetus of many species, including man (26, 27, 28). The relative impermeability of the placenta to other substances and the small capacity of foetal liver for gluconeogenesis (13) suggest that glucose of maternal origin may be the principal substrate for both lipogenesis and glycogenesis. Studies on the rabbit suggest that most of the foetal lipid is synthesized by the foetus (17) and foetal rat liver has a large capacity for lipogenesis from glucoce (29).

FOETAL GLYCOGEN RESERVES

The amount of lipid stored by the foetus varies enormously from species to species, but all species accumulate glycogen in the foetal liver and skeletal muscles. Except in the rabbit, the glycogen concentration in the foetal liver at term is about twice the usual adult concentration (Table 1). In species with a short gestation (rat, rabbit, dog, guineapig) the liver

Table 1. Foetal tissue glycogen concentrations at term in different species.

Species	Glycogen concentration (mg/g wet tissue)		
	Liver	Skeletal muscle	Cardiac muscle
Rat	90	11	27
Rabbit	40	15	14
Guineapig	70	18	3
Dog	115	18	15
Cat	–	–	13
Pig	85	72	15
Sheep	80	38	16
Monkey	90	30	10
Man	90 ?	30 ?	40 ?
Usual adult range	30–60	7–15	3–6

Reproduced with permission from Shelley (29a) by courtesy of the Nutritional Society.

glycogen remains low (< 5 mg/g) until a few days before term, but in other species the concentration begins to rise at a much earlier stage of gestation. In man the concentration has already reached 40–50 mg/g, the usual adult concentration by 20 weeks' gestation (30) and data from autopsy material (31) suggest that glycogen content continues to rise towards term. In all species the glycogen concentration in the skeletal muscles reaches adult levels early in gestation but, as shown in table 1, the concentration at term varies from ten times the adult concentration in the pig to four to five times the adult concentration in the sheep, monkey

and man, and near-adult levels in rodents and the dog. High concentrations
of glycogen are also present in the foetal heart. The concentration is about
ten times the adult level early in gestation, but later it usually falls and the
level at term (table 1) varies with foetal 'maturity'. It is high in the rat,
which is born naked, blind and relatively helpless, but has fallen to the
adult level in the guineapig, which is born looking and behaving like a
miniature adult. Man may be exceptional in that the high concentration of
early foetal life appears to be maintained right up to term.

To some extent the accumulation of foetal glycogen can be influenced
by nutrition. In rabbits the foetal liver glycogen concentration at term can
be lowered by chronic or acute restriction of the mother's food intake
(32, 33, 34), but the cardiac and skeletal muscle glycogen concentrations
are unaffected. Unusually low concentrations of glycogen in both the liver
and the skeletal muscles have been reported in several human babies of
low birth weight for gestation who died during the neonatal period (31,
35). The infusion of very large amounts of glucose (9 g/kg body wt.) to
pregnant rabbits during the six hours before delivery significantly raised
the foetal cardiac glycogen concentration but had no effect on foetal liver
glycogen (36).

The factors responsible for the changes in tissue glycogen concentration
at different stages of foetal development are not yet fully understood. In
foetal liver, the only tissue studied in detail, the activity of the enzymes
concerned with glycogen synthesis increases at about the time that glycogen begins to accumulate (37, 38). The changes in enzyme activity and
the rise in liver glycogen appear to depend on foetal pituitary and adrenal
function; both cortisone and a pituitary or placental 'growth hormone'
may be involved (39, 40).

THE FOETAL BLOOD GLUCOSE CONCENTRATION

There is general agreement that the foetal blood glucose concentration
varies with the maternal level, but there is some doubt about the exact
relationship between the two and whether this changes with gestational
age. A recent report by Goodner, Conway and Werrbach (41), states that
in the foetal rat the plasma glucose concentration rises during the last
three days of gestation from about 20 mg/100 ml (less than half the
maternal level) to equal the maternal level of 60–100 mg/100 ml at etrm.
Earlier work of the same authors was, however, criticized by Shelley and
Neligan (31) who attributed the occurrence of high foetal blood glucose
concentrations in late pregnancy to the mobilization of foetal liver glyc-

ogen. A large rise in blood glucose concentration in response to oxygen lack has been demonstrated in foetuses near term and in newborn animals of several species, but when the liver glycogen is low (as in early gestation), the blood glucose falls in anoxia (42, 43, 44, 45, 46, 34). By excluding all foetuses where there were signs of hypoxia, Shelley and Neligan (31) showed that the foetal blood glucose level in the sheep, rhesus monkey and rabbit remained at about half the maternal level right up to term. Since the normal maternal blood glucose level is about 40 mg/100 ml in the sheep and about 60 mg/100 ml in the rabbit and monkey, the materno-foetal glucose gradient was usually 20–30 mg/100 ml. Much larger gradients, 50–70 mg/100 ml, were reported by Shelley and Neligan (31) in rabbits where the maternal glucose level was high, but these observations were made in conditions where the maternal level was probably rising rapidly and it is likely that equilibrium had not been established between the maternal and foetal levels.

A materno-foetal glucose gradient of 20–30 mg/100 ml is also found in the majority of human babies at delivery (2). But the maternal concentration usually rises above 100 mg/100 ml in the second stage of labour and the levels of 70–100 mg/100 ml usually found in cord blood samples at vaginal delivery are unlikely to be representative of the normal foetus in utero. It is likely that the normal resting levels are nearer those found by Stembera and Hodr (2) at elective caesarean section, 75 mg/100 ml in the mother, 59 mg/100 ml in the umbilical vein and 53 mg/100 ml in the umbilical artery. Similar pre-labour values have been reported recently in women where blood samples were taken from the foetal scalp immediately after artificial rupture of the membranes (5). Foetal levels below 50 mg/100 ml at delivery, similar to those found in animal species by Shelley and Neligan (31), have been found in individual cases where the maternal level was low, and in situations where the foetal liver glycogen concentration was likely to be low, as in early pregnancy (47), in 'small for dates' babies and in some cases of antepartum haemorrhage (48).

The close relationship between the maternal and foetal blood glucose levels tends to obscure the fact that in late gestation the foetus is able to regulate its own blood glucose concentration to some extent. The mobilization of foetal liver glycogen in animals in response to hypoxia has already been mentioned and the observation that in severely asphyxiated babies the blood glucose concentration is often higher in the umbilical artery than in the vein (2a, 3) suggests that it occurs in the human foetus.

During late gestation the ability to release insulin in response to a glucose load also develops in both the human foetus and the foetal lamb (47, 19), though the response is sluggish compared with that of the adult (4). Recently Hoet (49) has attributed the insensitivity of the foetal pancreas to glucose to the relative constancy of the maternal (and hence the foetal) blood glucose level, and has suggested that the hypertrophy of the pancreatic islet tissue and higher resting levels of plasma insulin in the baby of the diabetic mother may be the consequence of wider fluctuations in the maternal glucose level. It is not known to what extent the foetal insulin level controls the uptake of glucose by the normal foetus, but it is tempting to attribute the high birth weight of many babies of diabetic mothers not only to the larger amounts of glucose which may be available to the foetus but also to the possible growth-promoting effects of the high foetal plasma insulin level.

GLUCOSE AND GLYCOGEN METABOLISM IN THE HYPOXIC FOETUS

The metabolic response of the foetus to hypoxia has been reviewed recently in some detail (50). Whereas there may be some doubt about the role of glucose metabolism in the normal foetus, there is no doubt of its importance in the hypoxic foetus, for in the absence of oxygen anaerobic glycolysis becomes the only major source of energy. If glycolysis is inhibited, the remarkable ability of foetal and newborn animals to survive anoxia is greatly reduced; a normal newborn rat a 24°C will survive for 50 min in 100% nitrogen but for only 3 min after pre-treatment with iodoacetate, no longer than the normal adult (51, 52). The prolonged survival of the untreated rats was partly due to hypothermia, but even at 36–38°C, temperatures nearer the normal intra-uterine environment, foetal and newborn rats will survive without oxygen for 20–28 min and foetal lambs in midgestation for a long as 40 min (53, 43, 42). This tolerance to anoxia is lost with increasing 'maturity' in both foetal and newborn animals, and that of lambs and guinea pigs at term is little better than that of adults.

The end point of anaerobic glycolysis is lactic acid and during anoxia large amounts of lactate accumulate in the blood and tissues of foetal and newborn animals. At first it was thought that the tolerance of newborn rats and mice to anoxia was due to an unusual capacity for glycolysis which was lost with advancing age (54), but as shown in figure 2, the rate of rise of blood lactate in anoxia appears to be a characteristic of the

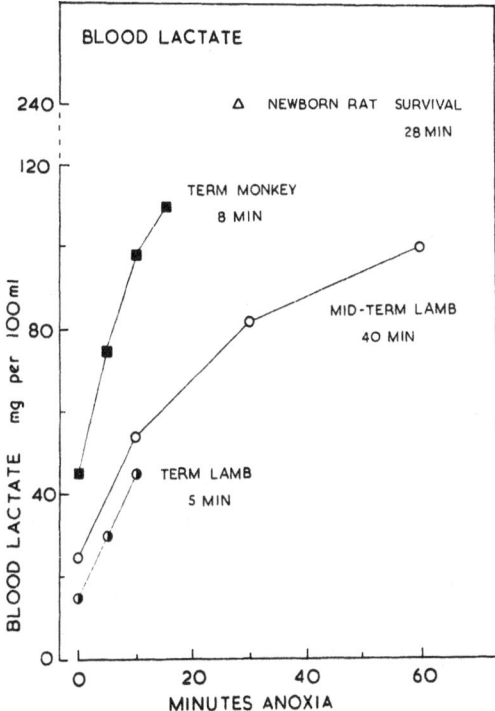

Fig 2 The blood lactate levels in foetal lambs in mid – (◯) and late (◐) gestation and foetal rhesus monkeys (■) asphyxiated by tying the umbilical cord, and in newborn rats (△) breathing 100% nitrogen. Their body temperatures were maintained at 35–38°C and their surival times are shown in parentheses. Data from Dawes et al. (42, 55), Dawes, Jacobson et al. (56), and Stafford and Weatherall (43) Reproduced from Shelley (50) by courtesy of the Journal of Obstetrics and Gynaecology of the British Empire.

species not of its stage of development. Certainly, the newborn rat has a phenomenal ability to produce lactate, the blood lactate rises to 240 mg/100 ml within 28 min, but the rate of rise in the foetal monkey, which survives undamaged for little more than 8 min, is considerably greater than that in the immature foetal lamb which survives for 40 min, even longer than the newborn rat. Moreover the initial rate of rise in the blood (and tissues) of lambs at term (survival time 5 min) is identical to that in the immature lambs and in adult ewes breathing 100% nitrogen (42).

This observation suggested to Dawes, Mott and Shelley (42) that anoxic survival might be limited not by the activity of enzymes in the glycolytic pathway, but by the amount of glucose or glycogen available to a vital organ such as the heart or brain. The glycogen content of the brain is low at all ages (27) but, as mentioned earlier, that of the heart is extremely variable and, within limits, is closely related to the ability to survive anoxia. For instance, the great tolerance to anoxia of the immature foetal lamb and the newborn rat is associated with cardiac glycogen levels of 25–35 mg/g (42), whereas in the newborn guineapig both the cardiac glycogen concentration and the anoxic survival time approximate to that of the adult. The cardiac glycogen is used by the cardiac muscle to provide energy for the maintenance of the circulation and its concentration falls rapidly in anoxia; when the initial concentration is low it is soon exhausted, but when it is high the circulation can be maintained for a relatively long time.

Maintenance of the circulation is essential for anoxic survival not only because it is needed to transport oxygen to the tissues when this is readmitted, but also because it is needed to transport glucose to glycogen-poor tissues such as the brain and to remove the products of glycolysis from the tissues during anoxia. The dependence of cerebral activity on the blood glucose supply was demonstrated by Stafford and Weatherall (43) who showed that in anoxic newborn rats the 'time to last gasp' was halved in insulin hypoglycaemia, although the initial cardiac glycogen concentration and the activity of the heart were unaffected. Conversely the gasping time could be prolonged by administering glucose to newborn rats from a litter where the liver glycogen had been exhausted and the blood glucose would have fallen during anoxia. Thus anoxic survival usually depends not only on the cardiac glycogen concentration but also on the liver glycogen; when this is present it is mobilized to provide glucose for the brain, and the administration of glucose to rats that are capable of raising their own blood glucose concentration does *not* prolong survival.

But the supply of glucose or glycogen is not the only factor limiting anoxic survival, for death usually occurs before the reserves have been fully depleted; even in the heart the terminal glycogen concentration may be 5 mg/g or more when the initial concentration is high. During anoxia there is a profound metabolic acidosis which is almost certainly due to the large amounts of lactic acid formed in the tissues. As shown in figure 3, the pH of the blood falls from about 7.4 to below 7.0 within 10–20 min in foetal and newborn animals at 36–38°C, and at the time of death it is usually below 6.8. As the pH falls, glycolysis is gradually inhibited until, when the arterial pH falls below 6.9, there is no further rise in blood or tissue lactate. Thus the acidosis, not the carbohydrate supply, becomes the factor limiting glycolysis and therefore survival.

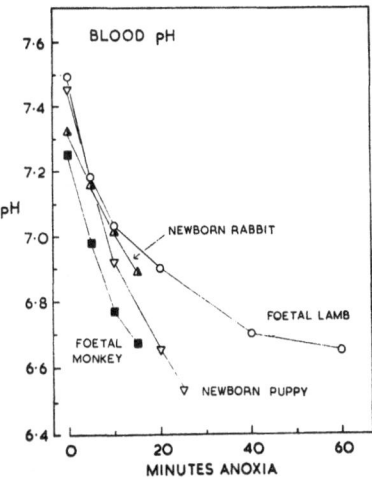

Fig. 3. The pH of the blood in foetal lambs in mid-gestation (◯) and rhesus monkeys near term (■) asphyxiated by tying the umbilical cord, in newly-delivered rabbits (▲) breathing 100% nitrogen, and in newborn puppies (△) breathing 95% nitrogen + 5% carbon dioxide. Their body temperature were maintained at 35–38°C. Data from Dawes et al. (42, 55), Dawes, Jacobson et al. (56), Dawes (54a), and Miller and Miller (54b). Reproduced from Shelley (50) by courtesy of the Journal of Obstetrics and Gynaecology of the British Empire.

These relationships were investigated more fully in foetal lambs in mid-gestation. At this age there is little liver glycogen and the blood glucose falls to zero in lambs asphyxiated by tying the umbilical cord. Dawes, Mott, Shelley and Stafford (55) compared the effect of infusing a base (sodium carbonate, Tris or triethanolamine), to maintain the arterial pH above 7.2 throughout the period of asphyxia, with that of infusions of glucose alone or glucose with base. Fig. 4 shows the effect of these infusions on the pH, blood lactate, heart rate and blood pressure of the foetal lambs. It is clear that although the heart rate appeared to be directly related to the pH in these experiments (fig. 4A and B), the administration of base alone or glucose alone was not effective in maintaining a high rate of glycolysis (fig. 4C) or halting the fall in blood pressure (fig. 4D). When base alone was given, the cardiac glycogen was completely exhausted and the lambs died of lack of carbohydrate; in lambs given glucose only, the acidosis inhibited glycolysis. But when glucose and base were administered together, a high rate of glycolysis could be maintained almost indefinitely (fig. 4C) and, after about 40 min, the blood pressure ceased to fall so rapidly (fig. 4D); one treated lamb recovered when the

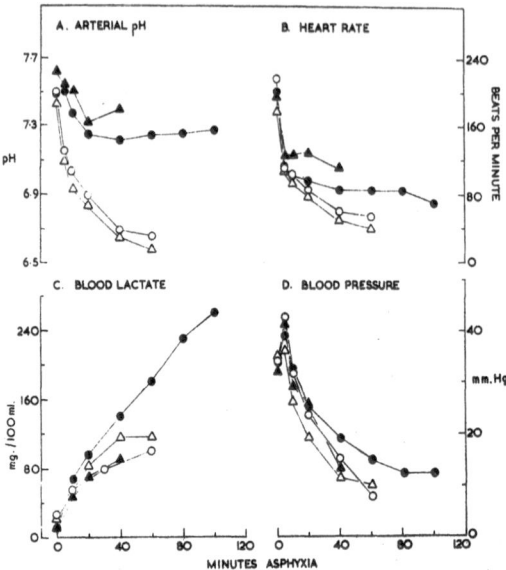

Fig. 4. The arterial pH (A), heart rate (B), blood lactate (C), and blood pressure (D) of untreated foetal lambs in mid-gestation asphyxiated by tying the umbilical cord (○), and of lambs receiving an infusion of sodium carbonate (▲), glucose (△), or sodium carbonate plus glucose (●) throughout the period of asphyxia. Data from Dawes et al. (55). Reproduced from Shelley (50) by courtesy of the Journal of Obstetrics and Gynaecology of the British Empire.

umbilical cord was untied after 80 min asphyxia, twice the usual survival time, and another still had a blood pressure of 10 mm Hg after 140 min asphyxia.

The infusion of a base with glucose had one other interesting effect (fig. 5). In the untreated lambs there was a steady rise in plasma potassium throughout the period of asphyxia; the initial concentration was about 4 mEq/l, and after 60 min asphyxia it was usually above 8 mEq/l. Giving glucose with sodium chloride or correcting the pH with a base alone had no effect, but when glycolysis was maintained with a base plus glucose, there was very little rise in plasma potassium. In the best experiment, where the blood lactate rose by nearly 200 mg/100 ml in 40 min, the plasma potassium rose by less than 0.5 mEq/l. This suggested that the maintenance of a high rate of glycolysis not only helped the heart to maintain the circulation, but also provided energy for the maintenance of tissue integrity; the rise in plasma potassium was almost certainly due to leakage from tissue cells and might therefore be taken as an index of cell dysfunction.

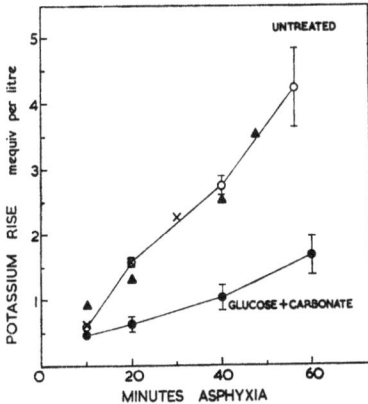

Fig. 5. The rise in plasma potassium concentration in untreated foetal lambs in mid-gestation asphyxiated by tying the umbilical cord (○), and in lambs receiving an infusion of sodium carbonate (▲), glucose plus sodium chloride (×), or glucose plus sodium carbonate (●) throughout the period of asphyxia. Redrawn with permission of the Journal of Physiology from Dawes et al. (55).

Support for this view came from later work on foetal monkeys. It was disappointing to find that when a base plus glucose was administered to foetal lambs or monkeys near term (56) their survival could be prolonged by only a few minutes, although the effect on glycolysis was similar to that in the immature lambs. The reason for this is probably that the rate of ATP utilization by many tissues increases during development (for references see 28); the rather slow rate of ATP production in anaerobic glycolysis may be able to keep pace with the rate of ATP breakdown early in gestation, but not at the relatively advanced stage of development of the foetal lamb and monkey at term. But there were strong indications that the treatment was of value in other ways. When rhesus monkeys near term are asphyxiated beyond the last gasp and are then resuscitated by tracheal intubation and positive pressure insufflation, characteristic lesions can be demonstrated in the brain stem nuclei when they are killed 1–2 months later (57). But when the monkeys were treated with glucose plus base during the latter part of the asphyxial period (58), they were easier to resuscitate and the amount of damage in the central nervous system was greatly reduced. In the two best experiments, where the arterial pH was corrected rapidly, there were *no* demonstrable lesions. It looked as though the infusion had completely protected these monkeys from anoxic brain damage even though treatment was not begun until after the onset of asphyxia, the situation which is likely to occur in clinical practice.

This discussion of the foetal response to hypoxia has been confined to animal species, for only in these it is possible to make unequivocal experiments on the effects of oxygen lack. But there is good evidence that similar changes do occur in the human foetus. In normal babies at delivery the blood lactate level is low, similar to that in the mother, and the umbilical arterio-venous difference is small, but in severely asphyxiated babies the blood lactate level in the umbilical vein may be 20 mg/100 ml or more above that in the mother, and the level in the umbilical artery may be 6 mg/100 ml or more above that in the vein (2, 2a, 3). The cardiac glycogen is usually grossly depleted in babies who die from asphyxial causes and the liver glycogen is also partially depleted (50). It is common knowledge that such babies are acidotic and the plasma potassium may be high. Moreover, there is increasing evidence that birth asphyxia may be associated with the development of neurological abnormalities not only in the monkey but also in man (59). It is likely that the high cardiac glycogen concentration and plentiful supply of liver glycogen in the human foetus will enable him to survive a fair degree of asphyxia, and it is to be hoped that his stage of development at birth is such that attempts to correct his acidosis and provide glucose to sustain him may be successful not only in ensuring survival but also in reducing the incidence of undesirable neurological sequelae.

REFERENCES

1. Widdas W. F., Transport mechanisms in the foetus. *Br. med. Bull.* 17, 107–111 (1961).
2. Štembera Z. K. and Hodr J., I. The relationship between the blood levels of glucose, lactic acid and pyruvic acid in the mother and both umbilical vessels of the healthy fetus. *Biol. Neonat.* 10, 227–238 (1966).
2a. Štembera Z. K. and Hodr J. II. Mutual relationships between the levels of glucose, pyruvic acid and lactic acid in the blood of the mother and of both umbilical vessels in hypoxic fetuses. *Biol. Neonat.* 10, 303–315 (1966).
3. Štembera Z. K., Hodr J. and Janda J., Differences in metabolism of healthy and hypoxic foetuses rated according to the arterio-venous difference in oxygen, glucose, lactic acid and pyruvic acid contents in the umbilical vessels and to the amount of blood flowing through the umbilical cord. In: *Intra-uterine dangers to the foetus,* pp. 77—83 (ed. J. Horsky and Z. K. Štembera). Excerpta Medica, Amsterdam 1967.
4. Thomas K., Gasparo M. de, and Hoet J. J., Insulin levels in the umbilical vein and in the umbilical artery of newborns of normal and gestational diabetic mothers. *Diabetologia* 3, 299–304 (1967).
5. Raivio K. O. and Teramo K., Blood glucose of the human fetus prior to and during labor. *Acta Paediat. Scand.* 57, 512–516 (1968).

6. Thalme B. and Engström L., Acid base and electrolyte balance in newborn infants of diabetic mothers. *Acta Paediat. Scand.* 58, 449–459 (1969).
7. Stembera Z. K., Hodr J. and Janda J., Umbilical blood flow in healthy newborn infants during the first minutes after birth. *Am. J. Obstet. Gynec.* 91, 568–574 (1965).
8. Scopes J. W., Metabolic rate and temperature control in the human baby. *Br. med. Bull.* 22, 88–91 (1966).
9. Alexander D. P., Britton H. G. and Nixon D. A., Observations on the isolated foetal sheep with particular reference to the metabolism of glucose and fructose. *J. Physiol., Lond.* 185, 382–399 (1966).
10. Britton H. G., Nixon D. A. and Wright G. H. The effects of acute hypoxia on the sheep foetus and some observations on recovery from hypoxia. *Biol. Neonat.* 11, 277–301 (1967).
11. Yarnell G. R., Nelson P. A. and Wagle S. R., Metabolism of gluconeogenic precursors in embryonic and fetal livers. *Fed. Proc.* 25, 449 (1966).
12. Yeung D. and Oliver I. T., Gluconeogenesis from amino acids in neonatal rat liver. *Biochem. J.* 103, 744–748 (1967).
13. Vernon R. G., Eaton S. W. and Walker D. G., Carbohydrate formation from various precursors in neonatal rat liver. *Biochem. J.* 110, 725–731 (1968).
14. van Duyne C. M., Parker H. R., Havel R. J. and Holm L. W., Free fatty acid metabolism in fetal and newborn sheep. *Amer. J. Physiol.* 199, 987–990 (1960).
15. van Duyne C. M., Havel R. J. and Felts J. M., Placental transfer of palmitic acid – 1 – C[14] in rabbits. *Amer. J. Obstet. Gynec.* 84, 1069–1074 (1962).
16. Koren Z. and Shafrir E., Placental transfer of free fatty acids in the pregnant rat. *Proc. Soc. exp. Biol. Med.* 116, 411–414 (1964).
17. Popjak G. and Beeckmans M. L., Synthesis of cholesterol and fatty acids in foetuses and in mammary glands of pregnant rabbits. *Biochem. J.* 46, 547–558 (1950).
18. Alexander D. P., Britton H. G., Cohen N. M. and Nixon D. A., Foetal metabolism. In: *Ciba Foundation Symposium on Foetal Autonomy* (ed. G. E. W. Wolstenholme and M. O'Connor), pp. 95–113. J. and A Churchill Ltd., London 1969.
19. Alexander D. P., Britton H. G., Cohen N. M. and Nixon D. A., Plasma concentrations of insulin, glucose, free fatty acids and ketone bodies in the foetal and newborn sheep and the response to a glucose load before and after birth. *Biol. Neonat.* 14, 178–193 (1969).
20. Pugh P. D. S. and Scarisbrick R., Acetate uptake by the foetal sheep. *J. Physiol., Lond.* 129, 67P (1955).
21. Alexander D. P., Britton H. G. and Nixon D. A., Metabolism of ketone bodies by the sheep foetus. *J. Physiol. Lond.* 186, 100–101 (1966).
22. Alexander D. P., Britton H. G. and Nixon D. A., Acetate metabolism in the isolated sheep foetus. *J. Physiol., Lond.* 190, 295–307 (1967).
23. Šabata V., Hahn P. and Drahota Z., The role of glucose and of keto-substances in the metabolism of foetuses of mothers suffering from diabetes. In: *Intra-uterine dangers to the foetus* (ed. J. Horsky and Z. K. Štembera), pp. 140–144. Excerpta Medica, Amsterdam 1967.
24. Šabata V., Wolf H. and Lausmann S., The role of free fatty acids, glycerol, ketone bodies and glucose in the energy metabolism of the mother and fetus during delivery. *Biol. Neonat.* 13, 7–17 (1968).
25. Britton H. G., Huggett A. St. G., and Nixon D. A., Carbohydrate metabolism in the sheep placenta. *Biochim. Biophys. Acta* 136, 426–440 (1967).

26. Widdowson E. M., Chemical composition of newly born mammals. *Nature, Lond.* 166, 626–628 (1950).
27. Shelley H. J., Glycogen reserves and their changes at birth and in anoxia. *Br. med. Bull.* 17, 137–143 (1961).
28. Dawes G. S. and Shelley H. J., Physiological aspects of carbohydrate metabolism in the foetus and newborn. In: *Carbohydrate Metabolism and its Disorders* (ed. F. Dickens, P. J. Randle and W. J. Whelan), Vol. 2. pp. 87–121. Academic Press, London and New York 1968.
29. Ballard F. J. and Hanson R. W., Changes in lipid synthesis in rat liver during development. *Biochem. J.* 102, 952–958 (1967).
29a. Shelley H. J., Carbohydrate metabolism in the foetus and the newly born. *Proc. Nutr. Soc.* 28, 42–49 (1969).
30. Villee C. A., The intermediary metabolism of human fetal tissues. *Cold Spr. Harb. Symp. quant. Biol.* 19, 186–199 (1954).
31. Shelley H. J. and Neligan G. A., Neonatal hypoglycaemia. *Br. med. Bull.* 22, 34–39 (1966).
32. Hafez E. S. E., Lindsay D. R. and Moustafa L. A., Effect of feed intake of pregnant rabbits on nutritional reserves of neonates. *Amer. J. vet. Res.* 28, 1153–1159 (1967).
33. Harding P. G. R. and Shelley H. J., Some effects of intra-uterine growth retardation in the foetal rabbit. In: *Intra-uterine Dangers to the Foetus.* (ed. J. Horsky and Z. K. Štembera), pp. 529–531. Excerpta Medica, Amsterdam 1967.
34. Shelley H. J. and Thalme B. Some aspects of lipid and carbohydrate metabolism in foetal and newborn rabbits. In: *Stoffwechsel des Neugeborenen. Ergebnisse eines Symposions über 'neonatale' Biochemie* (ed. G. Joppich and H. Wolf). Hippokrates-Verlag, Stuttgart. In press.
35. Shelley H. J., The energy supply of the foetus in normal and abnormal circumstances. In: *Perinatal medicine* (ed. P. J. Huntingford, K. A. Hüter and E. Saling). Thieme Verlag, Stuttgart. In press.
36. Gelli M. G., Enhörning G., Hultman E. and Bergström J., Glucose infusion in the pregnant rabbit and its effect on glycogen content and activity of foetal heart under anoxia. *Acta Paediat. Scand.* 57, 209–214 (1968).
37. Ballard F. J. and Oliver I. T., Glycogen metabolism in embryonic chick and neonatal rat liver. *Biochim. Biophys. Acta* 71, 578–588 (1963).
38. Kornfeld R. and Brown D. H., The activity of some enzymes of glycogen metabolism in fetal and neonatal guineapig liver. *J. biol. Chem.* 238, 1604–1607 (1963).
39. Jost A. The role of fetal hormones in prenatal development. *Harvey-Lect.*, Ser. 55, 201–226 (1961).
40. Jacquot R. and Kretchmer N., Effect of fetal decapitation on enzymes of glycogen metabolism. *J. biol. Chem.* 239, 1301–1304 (1964).
41. Goodner, C. J. Conway M. J. and Werrbach J. H., Relation between plasma glucose levels of mother and fetus during maternal hyperglycemia, hypoglycemia and fasting in the rat. *Pediat. Res.* 3, 121–127 (1969).
42. Dawes G. S., Mott J. C. and Shelley H. J., The importance of cardiac glycogen for the maintenance of life in foetal lambs and new-born animals during anoxia. *J. Physiol., Lond.* 146, 516–538 (1959).
43. Stafford A. and Weatherall J. A. C., The survival of young rats in nitrogen. *J. Physiol., Lond.* 153, 457–472 (1960).
44. Dawes G. S., Jacobson H. N., Mott J. C. and Shelley H. J., Some observations on foetal and new-born rhesus monkeys. *J. Physiol., Lond.* 152, 271–298 (1960).
45. Rink R. D., The effect of body temperature on asphyxial survival and anaerobic

glycolysis in the newborn golden hamster. (Mesocricetus auratus). *Biol. Neonat.* 12, 292–305 (1968).

46. Edwards A. V. and Silver M., The effect of asphyxia on the plasma glucose concentration in new-born calves. *Biol. Neonat.* 14, 1–7 (1969).

47. Obenshain S., King K., Adam P., Raivio K., Teramo K., Räihä N. and Schwartz R., Human fetal insulin response to sustained maternal hyperglycaemia. *Pediat. Res.* 3, 380–381 (1969).

48. Phillips L., Lumley J., Paterson P. and Wood C., Fetal hypoglycemia. *Amer. J. Obstet. Gynec.* 102, 371–377 (1968).

49. Hoet J. J., Normal and abnormal foetal weight gain. In: *Ciba Foundation Symposium on Foetal Autonomy* (ed. G. E. W. Wolstenholme and M. O'Connor), pp. 186–213. J. and A. Churchill Ltd., London 1969.

50. Shelley H. J., The metabolic response of the fetus to hypoxia. *J. Obstet. Gynaec. Brit. Emp.* 76, 1–15 (1969).

51. Himwich H. E., Bernstein A. O., Herrlich H., Chesler A. and Fazekas J. F., Mechanisms for the maintenance of life in the newborn during anoxia. *Amer. J. Physiol.* 135, 387–391 (1942).

52. Hicks S. P., Developmental brain metabolism. Effects of cortisone, anoxia, fluoroacetate, radiation, insulin and other inhibitors on the embryo, newborn and adult. *Arch. Path.* 55, 302–327 (1953).

53. Becker R. F., King J. E., Marsh R. H. and Wyrick A. D., Intra-uterine respiration in the rat fetus. *Amer. J. Obstet. Gynec.* 90, 236–246 (1964).

54. Reiss M., Das Verhalten des Stoffwechsels bei der Erstuckung neugeborener Ratten und Mäuse. *Z. ges. exp. Med.* 79, 345–359 (1931).

54a. Dawes G. S., *Foetal and Neonatal Physiology*, p. 147. Year Book Medical Publishers, Chicago (1968).

54b. Miller J. A., Jr., and Miller F. S., Interactions between hypothermia and hypoxia-hypercapnia in neonates. *Fed. Proc.* 25, 1338–1341 (1966).

55. Dawes G. S., Mott J. C., Shelley H. J. and Stafford A., The prolongation of survival time in asphyxiated immature foetal lambs. *J. Physiol., Lond.* 168, 43–64 (1963).

56. Dawes G. S., Jacobson H. N., Mott J. C., Shelley H. J. and Stafford A., The treatment of asphyxiated, mature foetal lambs and rhesus monkeys with intravenous glucose and sodium carbonate. *J. Physiol. Lond.* 169, 167–184 (1963).

57. Ranck J. B., Jr. and Windle W. F., Brain damage in the monkey, *Macaca mulatta*, by asphyxia neonatorum. *Exp. Neurol.* 1, 130–154 (1959).

58. Dawes G. S., Hibbard E. and Windle W. F., The effect of alkali and glucose infusion on permanent brain damage in rhesus monkeys asphyxiated at birth. *J. Pediat.* 65, 801–806 (1964).

59. Drage J. S. and Berendes H., Apgar scores and outcome of the newborn. *Pediat. Clin. North America.* 13, 635–643 (1966).

INTRAUTERINE PRESSURE AND THE HUMAN FOETUS

T. K. A. B. ESKES

The human foetus lives in a capsule filled with fluid of which the walls are made of contractile material. The contractile material, called the myometrium, is responsible for a fluctuating pressure which is superimposed upon the atmospheric pressure.

Pipe-lines meant for respiration and supplies are beautifully arranged in a small area in the capsule being the placenta and the umbilical cord. The capsule is connected via vital pipelines with the maternal capsule.

This well known anatomical model can be well compared with the Apollo flights so perfectly planned and reaching the final goal: the moon. Almost everything could be controlled: the capsule, temperature, pressure and astronaut-monitoring.

In regard to obstetrics, a few questions can be asked:

1. How far is process-knowledge?
2. Is process-control necessary?
3. If necessary, how far then is process-control?

Let us start with the first question: How far is process-knowledge?

In reviewing *pressure data of the uterine capsule,* many obstetricians and occasionally physiologists recorded intrauterine pressure in the past. Most of them used fluid filled balloons connected with a mercury manometer and a conventional lever.

Alvarez and Caldeyro-Barcia in Montevideo (1) and Bosch in Sankt Gallen (2) were the first to introduce the fluid filled open-tip catheter into the amniotic fluid, connected to a pressure transducer, pressure-amplifier and a recording apparatus. As could be proven later on in collaboration with Braaksma and Janssens in the Free University of Amsterdam (3), the advantage of an open-tip catheter is the pure hydrostatic pressure transmission to a Wheatstone bridge. A rubber membrane, as the wall of a balloon, has unknown properties of elasticity varying with temperature

28

and does not always give a predictable and reproducible transmission of the exact intrauterine pressure.

To investigate *the pressure in the myometrial wall* itself, the Montevideo group inserted microballoons with a volume of 0,02 ml into the myometrium. As you can see in figure 1, the so-called zero pressure is not mentioned in the upper two channels which are supposed to record the intramuscular or intramyometrial pressure. Only a pressure range of 30 mm Hg between two lines is noted, this in contrast to the lowest channel in which amniotic pressure is accurately recorded. From these records it was concluded, that the pressure values in the myometrium were three times as high as in the amniotic cavity.

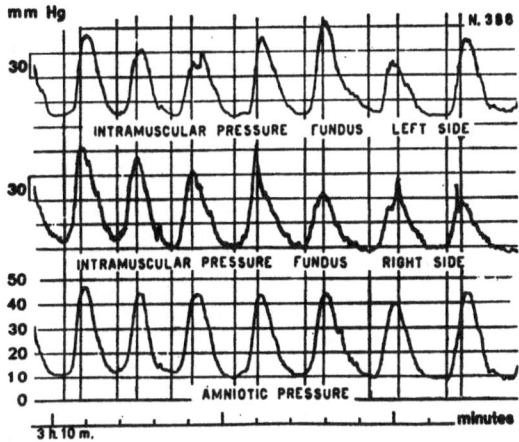

Fig. 1. Intramyometrial pressures (upper two channels) measured with microballoons in comparison with the intra-amniotic pressure measured with the open-end fluid filled catheter.
Note that intramyometrial pressures are approximately 2–3 times higher than the intra-amniotic pressure. (Reprinted with permission from Alvarez, H. and Caldeyro-Barcia, R.: Studies on the contractility of the pregnant uterus. *Proc. First World Congress on Fertility and Sterility.* New York, Intern. Fertility Assoc. 1953, p.p. 217–241).

In collaboration with Hendricks and Saameli in the Obstetrical Department in Cleveland (4) we inserted open-tip catheters in the myometrium. These catheters reflected pressures not three times higher than in the amniotic cavity, but almost equal or lower. In figure 2 the upper two channels reflect the pressure in the myometrium, the lowest channel gives the pressure of the amniotic fluid.

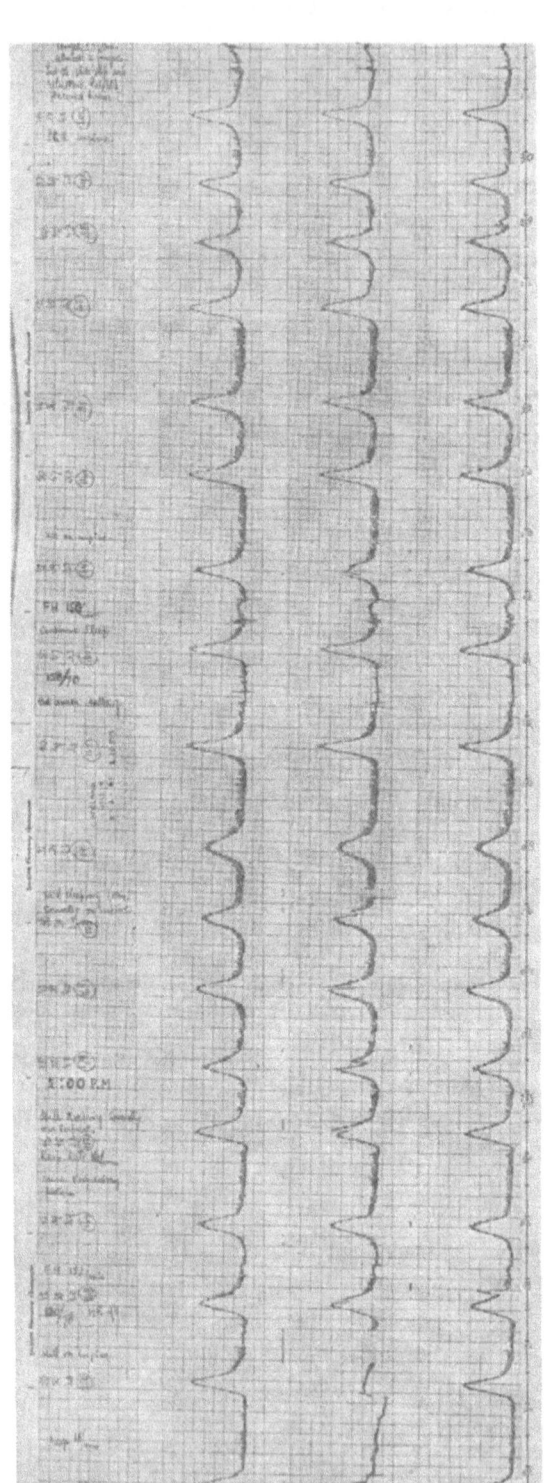

Fig. 2. Intra-myometrial pressures (upper two channels) and intra-amniotic pressure all measured with open-end fluid filled catheters. Calibration 0–100 mm Hg in all channels. Time-schale 3 blocks = 1 minute. Note that pressures are almost equal. Reproduced from Eskes (5).

This term pregnancy was stimulated with 40 nanograms/min of oxytocin, which equals 20 milli-units per minute. Due to placenta praevia, the location of the catheters could be chequed accurately during caesarean section. It could also be shown, that the inner layer of the myometrium reflected the amniotic pressure closely while a further gradient to the outer myometrial layer reaching values of the intraperitoneal pressure could be found (5) (fig. 3). Because of the fact, that also intervillous space pressures are closely related to the intra-amniotic pressure as demonstrated by Hendricks et al. (6), the pregnant uterus can be seen as a capsule in which pressures are homogeneously distributed.

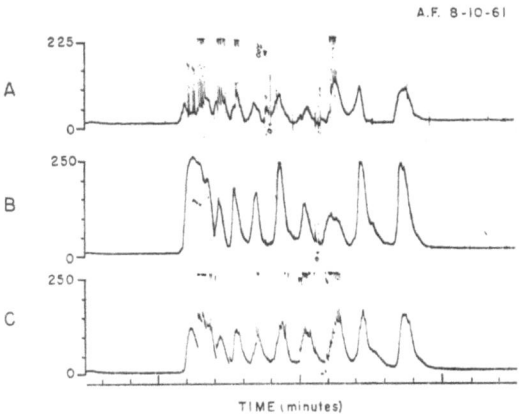

Fig. 3. Intramyometrial pressures in the postpartum uterus measured with open-end fluid filled catheters at different depth. A = superficial layer, B = deep layer, C = middle layer.
Note that a pressure gradient exists from the inner to the outer layer. Reproduced from Eskes (5).

These findings do have an impact on the concept of *the foetal and maternal placental circulation.* The umbilical vessels and their placental branches are located in a closed environment, so that superposition of intra-uterine pressure takes place. The myometrial vessels however, are in an open communication with the maternal circulation and will change their diameter if the transmural pressure, that is to say the pressure in the surrounding myometrium, exceeds the pressure in the lumen of the vessel (fig. 4).

Since intrauterine pressure values also during labour range from approximately 10–60 mm Hg, which will also be the value for intramyometrial pressure, it seems likely that compression of the venous channels in the myometrium already starts in the beginning phase of the uterine

T. K. A. B. ESKES

contraction, because the pressure in the caval system and its supplying channels is around 20 mm Hg. Also arterial compression is noted in the myometrium in the monkey studies of Ramsey et al. (7) and the studies in the human with radio-angiography of Borell et al. (8). Transmural pressure alone seems not to be responsible for this arterial compression because of the relatively low values for intrauterine pressure in relation to the intra-arterial pressure.

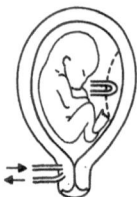

UMBILICAL VESSELS	UTERINE VESSELS
SURROUNDED BY A HOMOGENEOUS INTRA-UTERINE PRESSURE ENVIRONMENT GIVES SUPERPOSITION OF INTRAUTERINE PRESSURE	SURROUNDED BY CONTRACTING MYOMETRIUM WITH OPEN COMMUNICATION MYOMETRIUM LUMEN TRANSMURAL PRESSURE GIVES CONSTRICTION WHEN INTRAMYOMETRIAL PRESSURE EXCEEDS INTRALUMINAL PRESSURE

Fig. 4. Summary of the effects of intra-uterine pressure upon the 'closed' foetal circulatory system and the 'open' myometrial circulatory system.

When we summarize what happens during an uterine contraction we found:

- homogeneous pressure medium,
- no squeezing of blood from foetal villi to the main foetal circulation because of the closed environment the foetus lives in,
- some squeezing of blood from the uterus into the maternal circulation till venous occlusion occurs by transmural pressure,
- a myometrial gradient of pressure.
- a constriction of some arterial supply lines in radio-angiographic studies, perhaps meant to regulate the volume of the intervillous space,
- compression of the pelvic venous system and of the pelvic arterial system, commonly called the Poseiro-effect due to the heavy uterus in supine position in some cases.

What can be said about *the reactions of the foetal astronaut* on intrauterine pressure? Intrauterine pressure is usually measured and expressed in mmHg. If one translates that into centimeters of water, one places the foetus in the environment he belongs: water. When we continue this line of thought, the foetus can be seen as a swimmer on a level of approximately 10 mm Hg = 14 cm of water. This is presented in figure 5, where in the lower channel the intra-uterine pressure is measured in cm of water, as a mirror of the upper channel in which intrauterine pressure is recorded as usually.

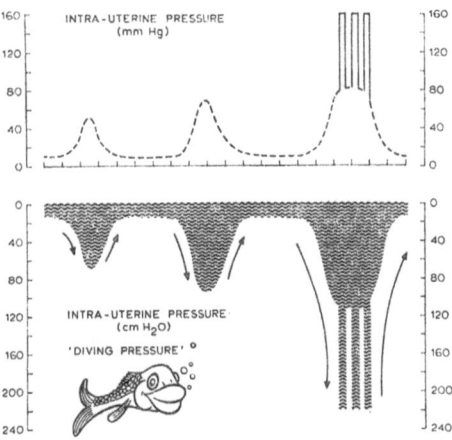

Fig. 5. Graph illustrating the foetus as a swimmer between uterine contractions and a diver during contractions to depths of 80 to 220 cm of water.

When the uterus contracts to a pressure of 60 mm Hg, the foetus has to dive to a depth of 82 cm of water or even deeper when the second stage with its super-imposed pushing pressure is reached. Also the bloodpressure of the foetus changes during this swimming and diving procedure.

In the pregnant monkey one can reach the foetal circulation without rupturing the amniotic sac. Due to the two placentas the monkey usually has, the communicating intraplacental vessels lying between the chorionic and the amniotic membrane can be reached and cannulated. In the upper channel of figure 6, you see the bloodpressure in such a vessel of a foetal monkey recorded simultaneously with the intra amniotic pressure in the lower channel. Although the calibration of both channels is different, a marked resemblance can be seen.

The reaction of the *foetal heart* can be much easier recorded. Scho-

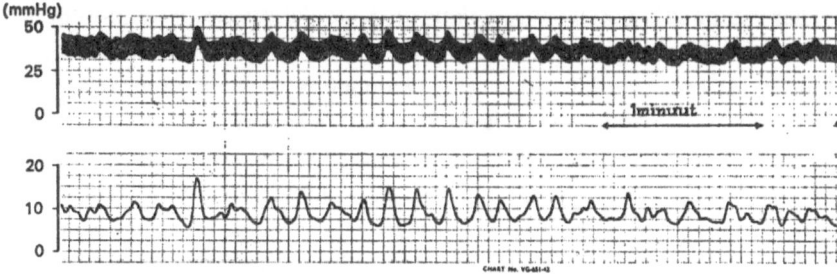

Fig. 6. Bloodpressure (upper channel) in a communicating vessel of the two placenta's of a foetal rhesus monkey with intact amniotic sac.

In the lower channel intra-amniotic pressure is recorded with a transabdominally introduced open-tip fluid filled catheter.

Note the resemblance between the two pressures during all phases of the uterine contractions.

lander (9) demonstrated that bradycardia occurred in seals during diving, which appeals to the slide in which we presented the foetus during labour as a diver. The foetal heart rate patterns are well described by Hon (10) and Caldeyro-Barcia et al. (11).

In figure 7 taken from Hon's compendium on this matter, foetal heart rate patterns are presented in relation to intrauterine pressure. In head compression an early deceleration of the heart rate pattern is seen, in utero-placental insufficiency a late deceleration is observed while the patterns in umbilical cord compression were variable.

We also used Hon's technic with indirect or direct leads (12). As you will expect, more factors are involved in the change of heart rate patterns than I showed you in the previous slide. One could list them as 'the diving procedure' of the foetus itself, the always complicated clinical entity of a patient, druginterference and so on. But as usual the method of recording, that is to say the method of integrating heartbeats in rate per minute, is essential for the patterns to be observed.

Thanks to our cooperation with the Medical Physical Institute T.N.O. in Utrecht, we could work with a beat to beat integrator. The records made so far in our team reveal more complicated pictures than the V- or U-dips or Type I and Type II dips described. It also made necessary to get *reduction of data.* Thanks to the work of Van Bemmel (13), Van der Weide and De Haan, the computer on line PDP-9 could be programmed for this purpose.

In figure 8 we show you tachograms of three different patients, in the first

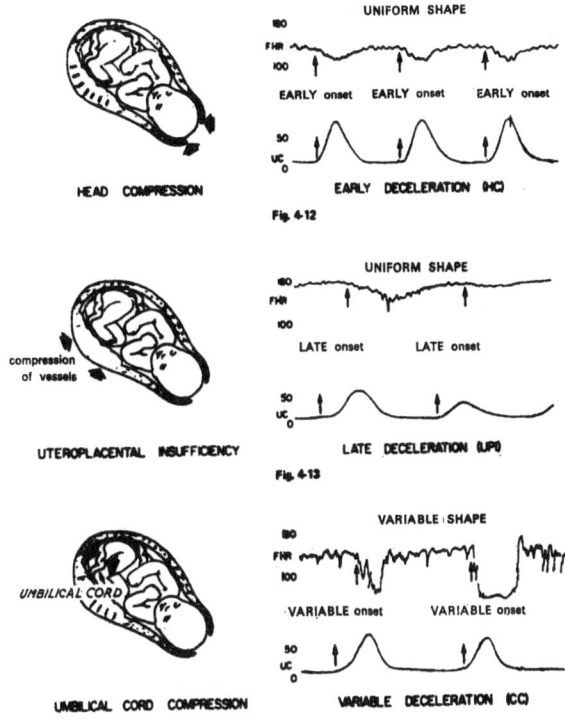

Fig. 7. Hon's classification of foetal tachograms in different clinical entities.

window of the upper row a tachogram is visible of approximately 4 minutes during labour. The duration of the intervals between two consecutive R-R-intervals is noted on the Y-axis, the time is noted on the X-axis. The distance between the clear points is 100 milliseconds. In the second window a differentiation is made between the 'angle' and the 'modulus'. The angle is the relationship between the consecutive heart beats, the modulus is the mean of consecutive intervals. The last one follows the heart rythm very closely in this case. The third picture of the upper row from the left shows a histogram composed of the first window, representing the intervals of the heart beats. The fourth window represents the histogram of the angle in the second window. The width of this diagram is a measure for the *short term irregularity*. The last window in the upper row is a histogram made from the last curve of the second window being the modulus and is a measure for the *long term irregularity*. If we follow the diagrams of the second patient in the second row, it is evident, that from the tachogram given in the first window the angle and the modulus in the

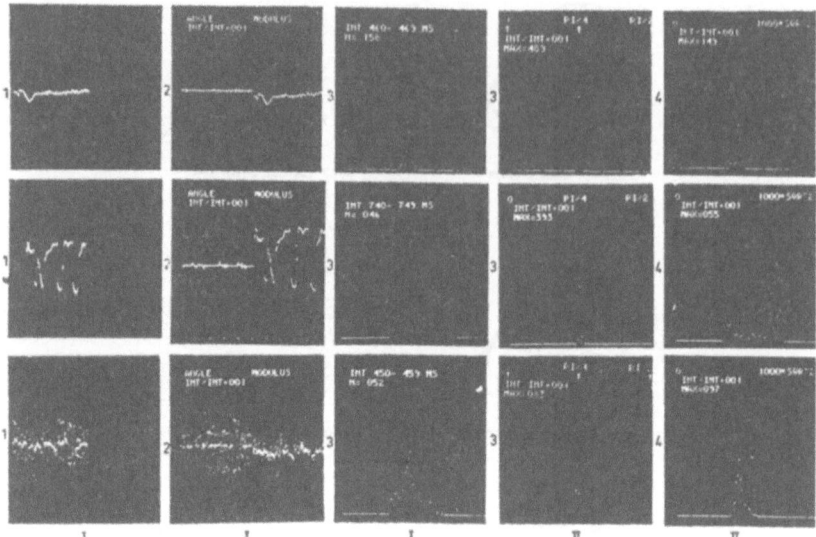

Fig. 8. Statistical evaluation of foetal tachograms (I 1) of three patients. Horizontal presentation.

The time is noted on the X-axis (distance between the clear points is 100 milliseconds), the duration of the R-R intervals is noted on the Y-axis (distance between the clear points is 100 milliseconds).

In the second window the angle (the relationship between the consecutive heart beats) and the modulus (the mean of consecutive intervals) is given.

The third window represents the intervalhistogram of the first window. The fourth window represents the histogram of the angle in the second window (a measure for short-term irregularity). The fifth window represents the histogram of the modulus (a measure for the long-term irregularity).

Note in the second row the small base of the fourth window (short-term irregularity) and the broad base of the fifth window (long-term irregularity).

Note in the third row the broad base of the fourth window (short-term irregularity) and the narrow base of the fifth window (long-term irregularity).

Reproduced from Van Bemmel (13).

second window differ markedly during an uterine contraction. The short term irregularity as noted in the fourth window is very much less than the long term irregularity in the fifth window.

In the third patient in the third row a very scattered tachogram can be seen. In the fourth window it is dinstinct, that the irregularity is due to very short fluctuations because of the broad base in the histogram in comparison with the narrow base on the fifth window indicating the long term irregularity.

To summarize: it is possible to define the term regularity or irregularity more precisely by computer evaluation and even to give a certain foetal trenddetection by means of reducing and processing data. We are very glad that the 'foetal heart project' as initiated by the engineers of the Medical Physical Institute and some of us, in which eight institutions in the Netherlands and in Belgium take part, cooperate in that way that even a division of tasks and projects was possible.

I still have two questions to answer: Is process control necessary and if so, how far is that control? I think we can control some of the process by interfering with uterine activity, for example in the stimulatory or inhibitory aspects or in the acute interference with the birth process by instrumental delivery.

Once Sikkel (14) and others said that approximately 70% of perinatal mortality and morbidity is related to pregnancy and labour. Maybe that it is true and gives the obstetrician a very heavy responsibility. The only plea we would make is to gather quantitative data to add to the already outstanding qualitative data in obstetrics we have. May be we then will reach the moon really!

REFERENCES

1. Alvarez H. and Caldeyro-Barcia R., *Surg. Gynec. Obstet.* 91, 1 (1950).
2. Bösch K., Inaugural Dissertation, Benno Schwabe & Co., Basel 1954.
3. Braaksma J. T., Janssens J. and Eskes T. K. A. B., *Europ. J. Obstet. Gynec.* (in press).
4. Hendricks C. H., Eskes T. K. A. B. and Saameli K., *Amer. J. Obstet. Gynec.* 83, 890 (1962).
5. Eskes T. K. A. B., *De druk in de menselijke uterus voor, tijdens en na de baring.* Thesis, Nijmegen 1962.
6. Hendricks C. H., Quilligan E. J., Tyler C. W. and Tucker G. J., *Amer. J. Obstet. Gynec.* 77, 1028 (1959).
7. Ramsey E. M., Corner G. W. and Donner M. W., *Am. J. Obstet. Gynec.* 86, 213 (1963).
8. Borell V., Fernström I., Ohlson L. and Wiqvist N., *Amer. J. Obstet. Gynec.* 93, 44 (1965).
9. Scholander P. F., In: *Oxygen supply to the human foetus.* (Ed. J. Walker and A. C. Turnbull) Blackwell, Oxford 1959.
10. Hon E. H., *Amer. J. Obstet. Gynec.* 77, 1084 (1959).
11. Caldeyro-Barcia R., Mendez-Bauer C., Poseiro J. J., Escarcena L. A., Pose S. V., Bieniarz J., Arnt I., Gulin L. and Althabe O., In: *The heart and circulation in the newborn and infant,* (Ed. D. E. Cassels) Grune & Stratton, New York 1966.
12. Eskes T. K. A. B., Seelen J. C., Stolte L. A. M., Van Bemmel J. H., Kuiper J., *Ned. T. Geneesk.* 109, 2369 (1965).

13. Van Bemmel J. H., *Detection and processing of foetal electrocardiograms.* Thesis Nijmegen, Utrecht 1969.
14. Sikkel A., De praeventie van cerebrale beschadiging van het kind tijdens de zwangerschap en baring. *Symposion B.O.S.K.,* 1967.
15. Caldeyro-Barcia R., In: *Physiology of Prematurity.* Transactions of the Fifth Conference. (Ed. M. Kowlessar) Josiah Macy Jr. Foundation, page 59, New York 1961.

FOETAL HEARTMONITORING AND BIOCHEMICAL EXAMINATION OF THE CHILD DURING LABOUR

R. H. GEVERS, P. E. R. RHEMREV AND J. FAVIER

Since January 1 1968 amnioscopy and microblood examination have been employed in the obstetrical department of the university of Leiden, using the Saling method (1), in all cases in which there is a possibility of a disorder in the foeto-maternal exchange. A disturbance of this sort can arise either during pregnancy or during labour. We list as potential disturbances in the foeto-maternal exchange:

A. *Disturbances during pregnancy*

1. toxaemia
2. dysmaturity
3. postmaturity
4. diabetes
5. bloodgroup antagonism

B. *Disturbances during labour*

1. meconium in the amniotic fluid
2. disturbances of the foetal heartrate
3. prolonged labour
4. disturbances during the second stage of labour

By means of employing amnioscopy and microblood examination where these disturbances occurred, in 1968 a drop was obtained in our perinatal mortality, and also a drop in our frequency of caesarean sections.

When, in 1969, we obtained access to the apparatus of the Institute of Medical Physics T.N.O. Utrecht which enabled us to record continuously the foetal heartrate and the foetal E.C.G., we wondered whether we would be able to obtain a further reduction in perinatal mortality and morbidity and whether this method of examination would indeed provide us with more and better information than the method of microbloodexamination.

We decided to combine both methods of examination. The women whom we wished to consider for this, were selected at the end of their pregnancy. Because the available apparatus and the thoroughness of the examination made it possible to keep only one woman 'under surveillance' at a time, our material is up till now based on only 33 cases. Of the pregnancies in question, 17 were normal and 16 were pathological pregnancies. Included in the 17 normal pregnancies were a few cases of postmaturity in which the amniotic fluid remained clear up to the time of birth, and in which the quantity of fluid was normal. The 16 pathological pregnancies were exclusively cases of: obvious toxaemia, dysmaturity, diabetes, severe Rh antagonism, and cases of postmaturity in which the amniotic fluid already contained meconium prior to labour.

EXAMINATION

a. Biochemical examination of the foetal blood:

pH O_2 saturation

pCO_2 glucose

Base Excess

Microbloodsampling was performed:

1. between 3–10 cm dilatation after rupture of the membranes (2–3 x)
2. on full dilatation
3. when head on the pelvic floor
4. in the umbilical artery and vena
5. 5 min., 10 min., 20 min., 30 min. and 60 min. after birth (not to be discussed here)

b. Continuous foetal heartmonitoring with scalp electrode, after artificial rupture of the membranes.

c. Continuous registration of the intrauterine pressure with open tip catheter, transcervical intra amniotic, after artificial rupture of the membranes.

a. *Biochemical examination*

The pH, pCO_2 and B.E. were determined with the aid of the Astrup apparatus and the Siggaard-Andersen-Engel normogram. The O_2 saturation was determined by the oxygen saturation meter type OSM 1 (Radiometer Kopenhagen). The glucose concentration was determined by the enzymatic bloodsugar estimation method with glucose oxydase and peroxydase (Boehringer Mannheim), modified by Reinouts van Haga. In table 1 the mean values are given.

Table 1. Mean normal values (Kubli) (2).

	First stage			Second stage		Umbilical artery
	0–2 cm	3–4 cm	5–10 cm	60–10 min.	10–0 min.	
pH	7,36	7,32	7,31	7,30	7,27	7,24
BE	–4,4	–5,6	–6,7	–6,7	–7,6	–9,1
pCO$_2$		44,5	46,3		49,9	51,9
O$_2$ sat.		34,7 ± 19,4			24,7 ± 16,3	22,7 ± 17

Mean normal values umbilical artery (Eckenhausen) (3):

pH   7,20
B.E.   –13
pCO$_2$ 41

In figure 1 the fall of the pH of mother and child during labour is illustrated according to Eckenhausen.

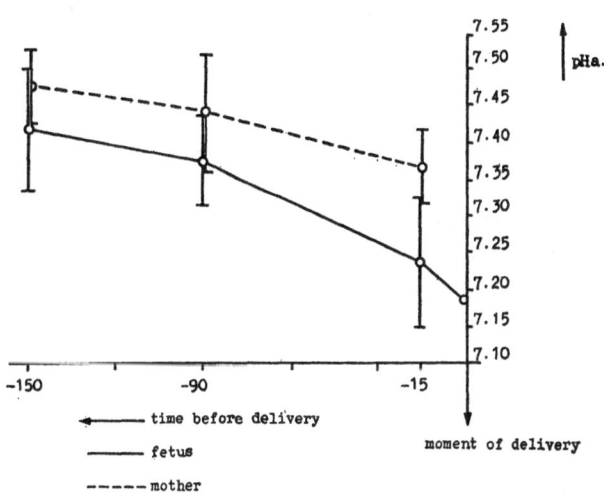

Fig. 1. Course of the actual pH of mother and child during labour until the
moment of delivery.

In the first 5–10 minutes after birth Eckenhausen (3) found a further fall
in pH of the child, followed by recovery in 1–5 hours, depending on the
condition of the child (fig. 2).

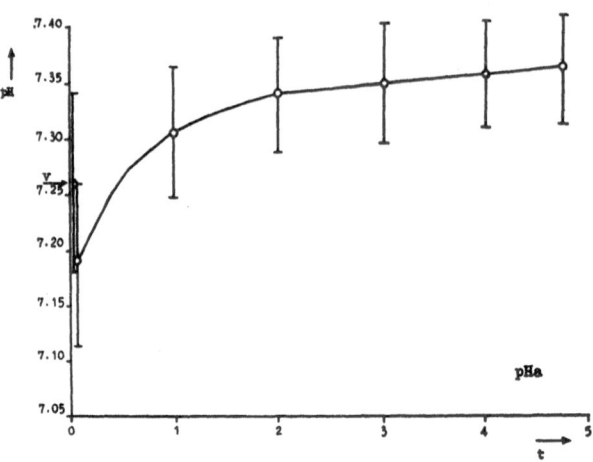

Fig. 2. Course of pH of mother and child after delivery.

b. *Foetal heartrate monitoring (F.H.R.)*
Hon (4) distinguishes 3 types of deceleration of the foetal heartrate:

1. Early deceleration, that is a deceleration of the foetal heartrate which coincides with a contraction of the uterus.
    This is said to be the result of headcompression (H.C.).
2. Late deceleration, that is a deceleration which is observed after the beginning of a contraction of the uterus. This is said to depend upon uteroplacental insufficiency (U.P.I.).
3. Variable deceleration, that is an irregular deceleration which begins at a different time from the contraction of the uterus. This is said to result from compression of the umbilical cord (C.C.).

The acceleration of the foetal heartrate is not discussed here.

On registering continuously the foetal heartrate and the contractions of the uterus, one is bound to wonder what form of bradycardia is still normal, and at what depth and what duration a bradycardia must be considered pathological. To answer this, Kubli, Hon, Khazin and Takemura (5) drew up the following criteria (see table 2).

Table 2. Principles of grading variable and late decelerations.

Criteria of grading	Mild	Moderate	Severe
Variabele deceleration			
Level to which F.H.R. drops and duration of deceleration	< 30 sec. duration, irrespective of level > 80 b.p.m., irrespective of duration 70–80 b.p.m., < 60 sec.	< 70 b.p.m., > 30 < 60 sec. 70–80 b.p.m., > 60 sec.	< 70 b.p.m., > 60 sec.
Late deceleration			
Amplitude of drop in F.H.R.	< 15 b.p.m.	15–45 b.p.m.	> 45 b.p.m.

The same authors divided the F.H.R. patterns into four groups according to their seriousness (see table 3).

Table 3. F.H.R. patterns and pH values.

Group	F.H.R. pattern	Mean ± S.D.	Averaged samples * (No.)
I	Variable deceleration (cc)–mild No deceleration Early deceleration (hc)	7.29 ± 0.046 7.30 ± 0.042 7.30 ± 0.041	42 71 16
II	Variable deceleration (cc)–moderate	7.26 ± 0.044	35
III	Late deceleration (upi)–mild Late deceleration (upi)–moderate	7.22 ± 0.060 7.21 ± 0.054	27 7
IV	Variable deceleration (cc)–severe Late deceleration (upi)–severe	7.15 ± 0.069 7.12 ± 0.066	10 10

* 218 averaged pH samples from 618 single pH samples.

At the same time, Kubli, Hon et al. (5) discovered a relationship between the group of the F.H.R. pattern and the pH of the foetal blood during labour, which is shown in figure 3.

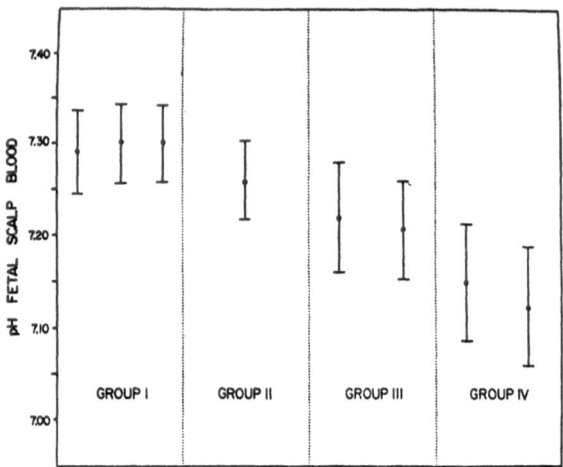

Fig. 3. Graph showing relationship between pH of fetal scalp blood and F.H.R. patterns (85 patients, 218 averaged pH determinations, 618 single pH determinations). Note four separate groups of mean pH together with the standard deviation for each category.

RESULTS

In our material we have divided the F.H.R. patterns into the same groups as Kubli, Hon et al. (5), and have compared this with the results of our biochemical examination. From this it appeared that in our material there was not a single case of group II.

So as not to burden you with too many figures, we give only the first values of pH, O_2 saturation and glucose in the first stage of labour, whereas we give the results of the examination of blood from the umbilical artery in full, because it is there that the condition of the child at the moment of birth is most clearly illustrated.

Our criteria for the term acidosis are based on the mean values which were discovered in our department by Eckenhausen.

In the normal pregnancies an oxytocine infusion was only administered when labour lasted too long. In the pathological pregnancies the oxytocine infusion was mostly administered in connection with pathology which had already been recognised by means of amnioscopy or microblood examination. It is therefore difficult to state with certainty whether the infusion itself contributed to worsening the pathology. This did however not appear to be the case in our material.

Table 4.

Normal group I

Birth w.	F.H.R.	pH I	pH art.	pCO$_2$ art.	B.E. art.	O$_2$ sat. I	O$_2$ sat. art.	Gl I	Gl art.	Ac	A.S.	Cord around neck	Part.
3600	normal	7,38	7,355	40,2	− 3,2	−	21	49	72	−	9	−	−
3450	mild C.C.	7,36	7,19	71,7	− 4,2	56	14	53	93	resp.	9	+	−
3420	tachycardy	7,44	7,28	36,1	− 9	−	22	88	91	−	7	++	inf.
3920	mild C.C.	7,43	7,145	41,1	−13,8	38	34	−	−	metab.	6	+	inf. Bracht
3810	mild C.C.	7,37	7,24	35,4	−10,1	66	29	41	59	−	8	−	−
2720	mild C.C.	7,41	7,19	70,7	− 6,3	48	30	−	−	resp.	9	−	−
4510	normal	7,34	7,28	49,5	− 4	63	53	−	−	−	9	−	−
3100	normal	7,31	7,20	127	−31	−	−	−	−	−	8	+	−
3410	normal	7,37	7,31	54,4	− 1,5	62	25	−	−	comb.	9	−	−
3100	normal	7,42	7,28	73,7		45	19	58	82	−	9	−	−
3600	mild C.C.	7,35	7,34	39,4	− 5	91	41	55	62	−	10	+	−

4 times acidosis of which 3 combined with encircling of the cord, A.S. 7 and 6 only in cases of prolonged labour.

Table 4 (continued)

Normal group III

Birth w.	F.H.R.	pH I	pH art.	pCO$_2$ art.	B.E. art.	O$_2$ sat. I	O$_2$ sat. art.	Gl I	art. Gl	Ac.	A.S.	Cord around neck	Part.
2790	mod. U.P.I.	7,28	7,22	48,8	– 9,8	72	32	43	62	–	9	–	–
3000	mod. U.P.I.	7,46	7,295	53,1	– 2,5	–	23	–	–	–	8	–	–
3100	mod. U.P.I.	7,42	7,22	77,8	– 3,8	–	17	53	69	–	9	–	–
3200	mild U.P.I.	7,38	7,355	62,9	– 3,7	63	11	77	74	–	9	–	inf.

No acidosis, no encircling, A.S. good.

Normal group IV

Birth w.	F.H.R.	pH I	pH art.	pCO$_2$ art.	B.E. art.	O$_2$ sat. I	O$_2$ sat. art.	Gl I	Gl art.	Ac.	A.S.	Cord around neck	Part.
2690	severe C.C.	7,44	7,15	95	– 3,9	42	8	47	66	resp.	9	–	inf.
3650	severe U.P.I.	7,26	7,255	70,7	– 5,3	62	55	56	117	–	8	–	inf. F

1 time acidosis, no encircling, A.S. good, cases of prolonged labour.

Table 4 (continued)
Pathol. group I

Birth w.	F.H.R.	pH I	pH art.	pCO_2 art.	B.E. art.	O_2 sat. I	O_2 sat. art.	G1 I	G1 art.	Ac.	A.S.	Cord around neck	Part.
2090	normal	7,40	7,31	40,5	– 2,7	78	22	86	153	–	9	+	inf. inverts.
2960	normal	7,315	7,24	40	–10,2	–	43	58	68	–	9	–	–
2140	normal	7,335	7,10	46,1	– 16,7	–	2	64	89	comb.	6	+	inf.
3940	normal	7,37	7,18	–	–	–	–	–	–	+ ?	8	–	inf.
3860	normal	7,31	7,19	58	–11,6	–	–	84	89	resp.	7	–	inf.
4000	normal	7,335	7,22	55,4	– 5,4	53	13	66	105	–	9	–	inf. F
3260	normal	7,255	7,16	50,2	–11,1	65	65	60	117	resp.	9	–	inf. VE

Some cases of acidosis, sometimes encircling.

Pathol. group III

Birth w.	F.H.R.	pH I	pH art.	pCO_2 art.	B.E. art.	O_2 sat. I	O_2 sat. art.	G1 I	G1 art.	Ac.	A.S.	Cord around neck	Part.
2810	mod. U.P.I.	7,33	7,29	37,6	– 7,7	32	32	–	–	–	8	–	inf.

Table 4 (continued)

Pathol. group IV

Birth w.	F.H.R.	pH I	pH art.	pCO₂ art.	B.E. art.	O₂ sat. I	O₂ sat. art.	G1 I	G1 art.	Ac.	A.S.	Cord around neck	Part.
1920	severe C.C.	7,375	7,16	75,6	– 6,7	79	15	61	67	resp.	9	+	–
3220	severe C.C.	7,29	7,13	77,2	– 8,8	64	20	76	92	resp.	8	+	inf.
1680	severe U.P.I.	7,25	7,12	–	–	–	–	–	–	+ ?	6	+	inf.
3680	severe C.C.	7,28	7,075	96,3	–11,4	48	13	49	100	resp.	4	+	inf. V.E.
2050	severe C.C.	7,31	7,17	51,8	–15,4	–	–	–	–	comb.	7	+	–
3550	severe C.C.	7,31	6,82	88,4	–22,9	30	5	–	–	comb.	4	++	–
2530	severe U.P.I.	7,295	7,22	29	–14,7	49	4	58	96	–	1	–	inf.
3110	severe U.P.I.	7,315	7,12	62	– 9,4	–	23	54	111	resp.	7	–	inf.

Nearly always acidosis and encircling, only 2 cases of good A.S., often low birthweight.

In the figures 4, 5 and 6 we give the average fall in the pH and the O_2 saturation, and the average rise of the glucose content in the foetal blood in the normal and the pathological cases.

It is evident that in the pathological group the pH begins, on average,

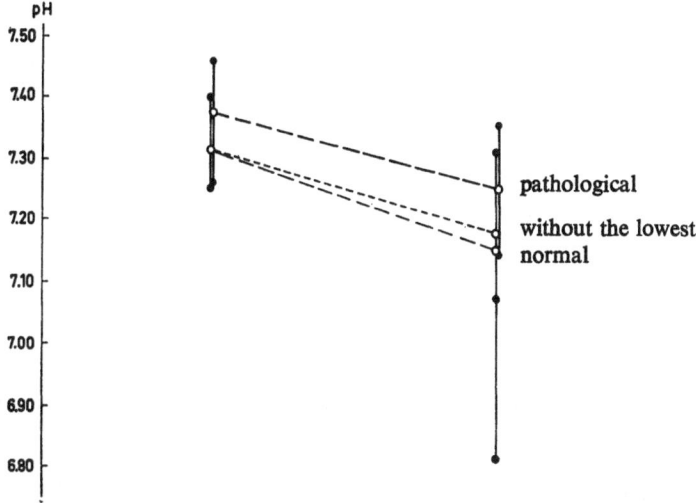

Fig. 4. Average fall in the pH in foetal blood in normal and pathological cases.

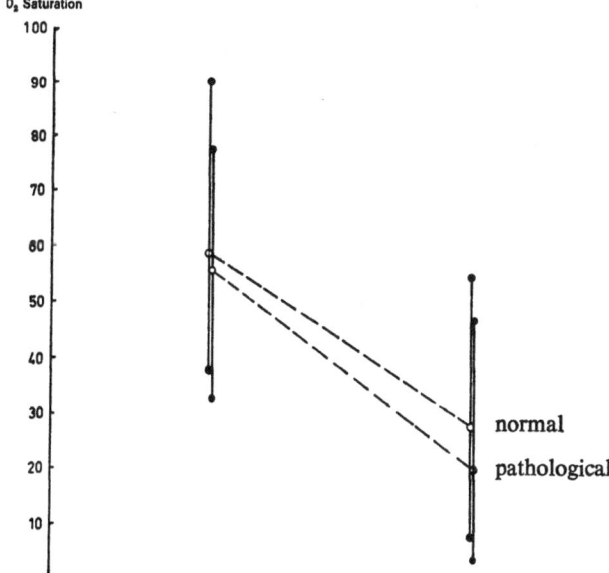

Fig. 5. Average fall in the O_2 saturation in foetal blood in normal and pathological cases.

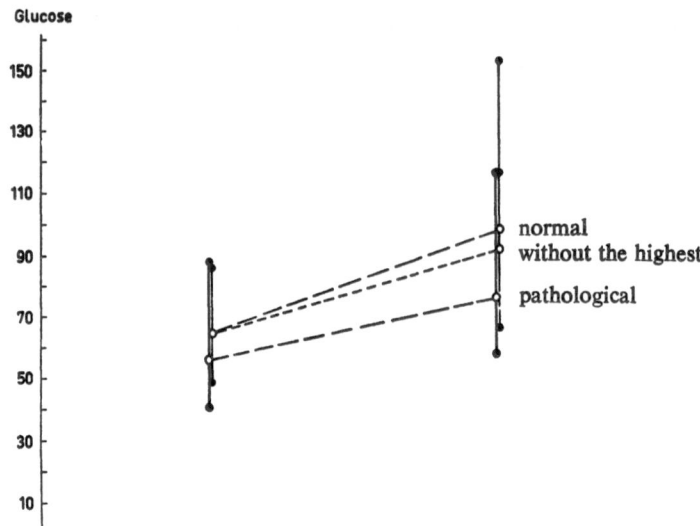

Fig. 6. Average rise of the glucose content in foetal blood in normal and pathological cases.

lower, and falls more, and that the glucose content begins higher and rises more than in the normal group.

In the case of the O_2 saturation, on the other hand the difference between the normal and the pathological group is much smaller.

The tables 5 a–d show the relationship between the groups of F.H.R. patterns, acidosis in the umbilical artery (pH < 7,20), Apgar Score 1 minute after birth, encircling of the cord round the neck and other particulars. The Apgar score was always exactly established by the same doctor.

From our examination it thus appears that:

– a good F.H.R. pattern without acidosis occurs frequently in the normal group and less frequently in the pathological group.

– a bad F.H.R. pattern without acidosis occurs fairly frequently in the normal group and seldom in the pathological group.

– a good F.H.R. pattern with acidosis occurs with equal frequency in both groups, the A.S. in these groups is not always optimal, and encircling of the cord occurs perhaps a little more frequently.

– a bad F.H.R. pattern with acidosis occurs in only one case in the normal group, but much more frequently in the pathological group. Moreover, the A.S. is usually decidedly too low, while encircling of the cord almost always occurs.

Table 5a

Good F.H.R. without acidosis	A.S.	Cord around neck	Part.
normal			
I	9	–	–
I	7	++	inf.
I	8	–	–
I	9	–	–
I	9	–	–
I	9	–	–
I	10	+	–
pathol.			
I	9	+	inf.
I	9	–	–
I	9	–	inf. F

Table 5b

Bad F.H.R. without acidosis	A.S.	Cord around neck	Part.
normal			
III	9	–	–
III	8	–	–
III	9	–	–
III	9	–	inf.
IV	8	–	inf. F
pathol.			
III	8	–	inf.
IV	1	–	Rh. inf. Plac. index 26

In the groups without acidosis one case was found of an A.S. 1, where there was a very serious Rh antagonism. The Hb content of the child was 3 g% and the placenta index was 26. And once an A.S. 7 was found, in a case of the cord being wound twice around the neck.

In the groups with acidosis there are 8 cases of A.S. 7 or lower. 7 of these were pathological pregnancies, whereas one was a normal pregnancy but with a prolonged labour and the child in breech presentation. Time and again we are struck by the fact that in the groups with acidosis, encircling

Table 5c

good F.H.R. with acidosis		A.S.	Cord around neck	Part.
normal				
I	resp.	9	+	
I	metab.	6	+	inf. prol. labour, Bracht
I	resp.	9	–	
I	comb.	8	+	
pathol.				
I	comb.	6	+	inf.
I	comb. ?	8	–	inf.
I	resp.	7	–	inf.
I	resp.	9	–	inf. V.E.

Table 5d

Bad F.H.R. with acidosis		A.S.	Cord around neck	Part.
normal				
IV	resp.	9	–	inf.
pathol.				
IV	resp.	9	+	
IV	resp.	8	+	inf.
IV	comb. ?	6	+	inf.
IV	resp.	4	+	inf. V.E.
IV	comb.	7	+	
IV	comb.	4	+ +	
IV	resp.	7	–	inf.

around the neck occurs more frequently than in the groups without acidosis. We saw it 10 times in the groups with acidosis and 3 times in the groups without acidosis.

Table 6 shows the relationship in the 8 cases mentioned with A.S. 7 or lower, between the F.H.R. pattern, A.S. and fall in pH.

Table 6

Normal or pathol.	F.H.R.	Group	Cord around neck	A.S.	pH I	pH art.	Sort of Acidosis
pathol.	I	norm.	−	7	7,31	7,19	resp.
pathol.	IV	severe C.C.	+	7	7,31	7,17	comb.
pathol.	IV	severe U.P.I.	−	7	7,31⁵	7,12	resp.
normal	I	mild C.C.	+	6	7,43	7,14⁵	metab.
pathol.	IV	severe U.P.I.	+	6	7,25	7,12	comb.
pathol.	I	norm.	+	6	7,33⁵	7,10	comb.
pathol.	IV	severe C.C.	+	4	7,28	7,07⁵	resp.
pathol.	IV	severe C.C.	+ +	4	7,31	6,82	comb.

In this table it is evident that the A.S. is correspondingly lower as the pH of the umbilical artery is lower.

We also went into the question of how often the pH from the umbilical artery is lower than 7,20, when the A.S. is 8 or higher. This can be seen in table 7.

Table 7

Normal or pathol.	F.H.R.	Group	Cord around neck	A.S.	pH I	pH art.	Sort of Acidosis
normal	I	mild C.C.	+	9	7,36	7,19	resp.
normal	I	mild C.C.	−	9	7,41	7,19	resp.
normal	IV	severe C.C.	−	9	7,44	7,15	resp.
pathol.	I	norm.	−	9	7,25⁵	7,16	resp.
pathol.	IV	severe C.C.	+	9	7,37⁵	7,16	resp.
pathol.	I	norm.	−	8	7,37	7,18	?
pathol.	IV	severe C.C.	+	8	7,29	7,13	resp.

It is obvious that in these cases the pH is not as far below 7,20 as in the cases where the A.S. is 7 or lower.

From these tables it appears that the value of the A.S. and the pH value of blood from the umbilical artery run pretty well parallel, but that the relationship with the F.H.R. pattern is less clear.

Finally we give in figure 7 the relationship between the pH of the umbilical artery and the seriousness of the F.H.R. decelerations, corresponding to the groups of Kubli, Hon et al. (5).

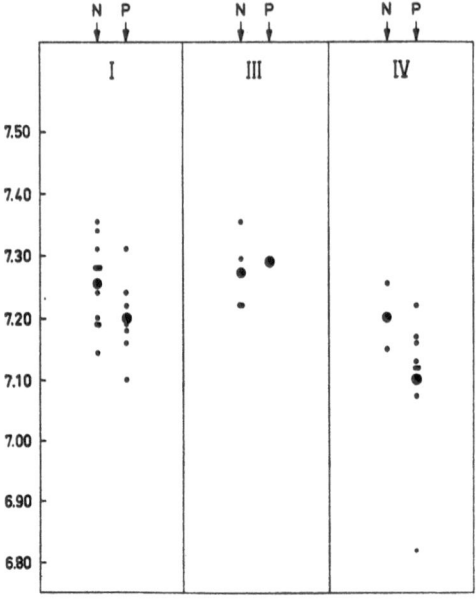

Fig. 7.   N = normal   P = pathological

Thus it appears that our pH values are, on average, lower than those of Kubli, Hon et al. (5), which can be explained by the fact that we used blood from the umbilical artery, whereas Kubli, Hon et al. gave the pH values during labour. In our material it is also evident that in the groups I and IV the pH values of pathological pregnancies were, on average, lower than in normal pregnancies.

DISCUSSION AND CONCLUSIONS

Although our material is still too small for final conclusions to be drawn, our provisional conclusions are as follows.

Foetal heartmonitoring with scalp electrode provides very good information about the foetal heartrate, but must be combined with internal measurement of the intra uterine pressure, because the information is otherwise inadequate. The F.H.R. pattern and the foetal E.C.G. can be registered continuously as soon as there is any dilatation, but a disadvantage of this method is, that it involves rupturing the membranes. The apparatus is expensive, and the method does not economise on personnel. Information is obtained only about the heart, but not about the child. Acidosis is repeatedly found even where the F.H.R. pattern is good, and no acidosis where the F.H.R. is bad.

The microbloodexamination can be frequently repeated, but for this, too, the membranes must be ruptured. The apparatus is less costly and this method does not require more personnel. When properly used it gives reliable information about the condition of the child. Almost all children without acidosis were born with a good A.S. even where the F.H.R. pattern was bad. The children with acidosis were often born with a poor or bad A.S., even where the F.H.R. pattern was good.

The combination of a bad F.H.R. pattern (group IV) with acidosis and an A.S. which is not optimal, or is bad, occurs almost exclusively in pathological pregnancies. There is a clear relationship between A.S. and pH of the umbilical artery, but the relationship with the F.H.R. pattern is not clear.

We would like, therefore, to offer the following advice: one must learn to make a sharp distinction, during prenatal care, between normal and pathological pregnancies. In all pathological pregnancies the child must be kept under surveillance with microbloodexamination during labour. If this is done, foetal heartmonitoring can be left on one side all together. In normal pregnancies, surveillance by means of microbloodexamination during labour is only indicated if meconium appears, or if the foetal heartbeats are not optimal, and always in prolonged labour or where there are disturbances during the second stage. Thus the grounds for continuous registration of the foetal heartbeats would seem to be extremely small in an obstetric department which is functioning properly. If on the other hand, one should wish to employ the method of foetal heartmonitoring, then preference should be given to confinements which have been preceded by normal pregnancies. Where a pathological F.H.R. pattern is found, a microblood examination is then indicated. It is, however, clear that the high cost of the apparatus is out of all proportion to the small return.

The significance of encircling around the neck is also clear to see from our material. In the groups with acidosis encircling occurs considerably more frequently than in the groups without acidosis. Encircling around the neck occurs most in the group of pathological pregnancies with a bad F.H.R. pattern (group IV) and acidosis. Thus the impression we obtain is that in pathological pregnancies, encircling around the neck is a far more serious complication than in a normal pregnancy, and can, of course, be 'the last straw, which breaks the camel's back'. It has been queried whether the distinction between C.C. and U.P.I. is in fact valid. In our material this does seem to be the case: in the pattern of C.C., encircling of the neck does indeed occur with conspicuous frequency. The pattern of U.P.I. does also occur in normal pregnancies, where there is no encircling of the neck.

It is also striking that the pattern of C.C. and of U.P.I. is seen most often in the case of children weighing less than 3250 gram, that is, smaller children. This corresponds to the view that a small placenta is more likely to be insufficient than a large one.

REFERENCES

1. Saling E., *Das Kind im Bereich der Geburtshilfe*. Thieme, Stuttgart 1966.
2. Kubli F., *Foetale Gefahrenzustände und ihre Diagnose*. Thieme, Stuttgart 1966.
3. Eckenhausen F. W., *A study of the perinatal acid-base equilibrium*. Thesis, Leiden 1969.
4. Hon E. H., *Am. J. Obst. Gynec.* 77, 1084 (1959).
5. Kubli F., Hon E. H., Khazin A. F., Takemura H., *Amer. J. Obst. Gynec.* 104, 1190 (1969).

IATROGENIC FETAL HYPOXIA

F. KUBLI AND H. RÜTTGERS

Iatrogenic diseases are defined as diseases due to medical interference. They must be as old as medicine itself. Their particular and almost tragic pecularity is given by the fact that measures taken to improve the health of human beings finally exert an opposite effect and are the cause of a new disease.

In obstetrics and gynecology the most famous example of iatrogenic damage is adverse influence on early development of the fetus by application of certain drugs to the mother in early pregnancy.

Concerning late pregnancy it is well-known today that several operative obstetrical procedures that were currently applied a few years ago – e.g. internal version, high forceps delivery etc. – were potentially dangerous to the fetus. Nowadays these are obsolete procedures which do not deserve any discussion any more. In the present paper we prefer to discuss some aspects of obstetrical attitudes and measures that are in current use and whose effect on the fetus is not adverse in a clearcut way but at most controversial. Some observations therefore will be presented on the following subjects:

1. Oxytocin augmentation of labor
2. Paracervical anesthesia
3. Possible adverse effects on the fetus caused by the fetal monitoring procedures themselves.

GENERAL REMARKS CONCERNING METHODOLOGY

The results presented are to some extent 'fall out products' of a six month's period of fetal intensive care performed at the Department of Obstetrics and Gynecology, University Clinics Frankfurt a.M. from January 15th 1969 to July 15th 1969. During this time the intention was to continuously monitor fetal heart rate and intrauterine pressure in all patients admitted to the labor- and delivery floor. The eventual yield of monitored fetuses, however, was 40% only, a total of about 300 patients. The findings of the FHR-records and fetal blood-gas analyses were compared in retrospect with some clinical data. This study on iatrogenic fetal hypoxia therefore is a clinical and retrospective study with all disadvantages and fallacies bound to this type of study.

In all cases fetal monitoring was done according to the method of Hon i.e. recording of instantaneous fetal heart rate on the basis of fetal electrocardiograms obtained by direct fetal electrocardiography (scalp electrode) and of intrauterine pressure transmitted by a transcervically inserted open-end-catheter to a Statham pressure transducer. Commercially available monitoring equipment was used – most often the Hewlett Packard Clinical Monitor 8020-A, in a minority of patients the Corometrics Clinical Monitor FMS-101. Fetal acid base balance and fetal pO_2 was routinely determined in umbilical cord-blood and less often – on clinical indication – in micro-bloodsamples during labor.

Fetal hypoxia in this study was defined as impairment of fetal oxygenation. This situation was thought to be present with the occurrence of certain abnormal fetal heart rate patterns and/or acidemia in fetal blood. Admittedly both, fetal heart rate patterns and fetal pH are subject to some controversy regarding their role as parameters of fetal hypoxia. However, a relativly large body of evidence has been accumulated demonstrating the relationship between abnormal fetal heart rate patterns and abnormal fetal acid base balance (1, 2) on the one hand, and between abnormal fetal acid base balance and clinical signs of hypoxia in the newborn on the other hand (3, 4, 5). It seems justified, therefore, in a clinical study on the human fetus, to take these parameters as indicative of impairment of fetal oxygenation and, in a clinical sense, of fetal hypoxia.

I. EFFECT OF CONTINUOUS INTRAVENOUS OXYTOCIN ON UTERINE ACTIVITY AND ON THE FETUS

Patients and methods

In 75 patients labor was either induced or augmented by oxytocin. Oxytocin was applied as intravenous drip. 3 Units of oxytocin were disolved in 500 ml of glucose. 20 Drops of the solution therefore correspond to 6 mU. Data concerning fetal heart rate, fetal acid base balance and uterine activity were compared with those of a reference group of 85 patients with spontaneous labor. This reference group was randomly selected from the rest of the monitored patients.

In both groups of patients frequency of uterine contractions for each period of 10 minutes as well as intensity of each contraction and the basal tone of each interval was measured. A total of about 9.000 contractions were processed in this way.

Both groups of patients are comparable concerning the total time during which their labors were monitored (about 160 hours in each group). However they are not comparable concerning parity and pregnancy complications, the oxytocin-group exhibiting a larger number of primigravida and of pregnancy complications than the control group. Evidently labor was not comparable for both groups, since oxytocin was given on clinical indications only.

Results

a. *pH in umbilical artery blood:* In table 1 mean fetal pH in umbilical artery blood in both groups is demonstrated. Fetal umbilical artery pH in the oxytocin stimulated group is significantly lower than in the control group. This difference might be due either to the effect of the oxytocin medication or to the differences in patient material.

b. *Definition and incidence of uterine hyperactivity*

ba. *Uterine hyperactivity as defined on a purely statistical basis:* In this study the definition of normal and abnormal labor has proved to be difficult because of two reasons:

1. The quality of uterine contractions changes with progressing labor as has been shown by Caldeyro (6), Cibils and Hendricks (7) and others years ago and
2. Even in spontaneous labor episodes of uterine hyperactivity may be observed.

Table 1. Mean fetal arterial pH in patients with and without oxytocin stimulated labor.

	n	pH Fetal Umbilical Artery X ± S
with oxytocin	65*	7.211 ± 0.066
without oxytocin	77*	7.250 ± 0.073
	p < 0.005	

* In 10 of the 75 patients with oxytocin and in 8 of the 85 patients without oxytocin umbilical artery pH was not available.

The first point is demonstrated in figure 1. Here the frequency distribution of basal tone values is shown for three given stages of cervical dilatation. These data were collected in a relatively small group of patients with known and comparable stages of cervical dilatation, and during a period of only 10 minutes for each patient and each stage of cervical dilatation. It can be shown that mean and upper range of basal tone is increasing with progressing labor. The upper limits are 14 mm Hg in early labor, 18 mm Hg in the late first stage and reaches a maximum of about 20 mm Hg at full dilatation. A statistically significant difference is found for mean

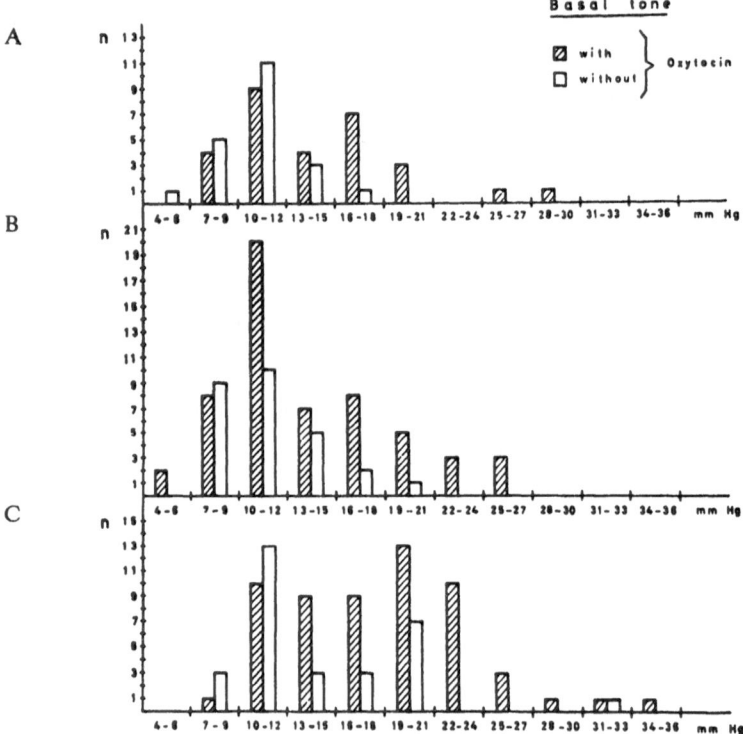

Fig. 1. Frequency distribution of basal tone values at different stages of cervical dilatation.
A. Cervical dilatation 3–5 cm. Number of patients without oxytocin 21, with oxytocin 29.
B. Cervical dilatation 6–8 cm. Number of patients without oxytocin 27, with oxytocin 56.
C. Full cervical dilatation (second stage of labor). Number of patients without oxytocin 30, with oxytocin 58.
n = number of patients.

basal tone at each stage of dilatation between the oxytocin group and the control group. However, it was felt that this approach did not give a true picture of the real situation, since in this way a small percentage only of all data is evaluated. In view of the fact that the results found in this small particular study group are very similar to those found by Caldeyro-Barcia and Kraphol (8) it was decided to accept the upper limits found in this small group during the late first stage as the overall upper limits for normal labor during the whole first stage irrespective of the exact stage of cervical delatation and to evaluate all recorded contractions against this reference data, e.g. 18 mm Hg for basal tone. The result, again for basal tone, is shown in figure 2. This figure demonstrates the frequency distribution of all basal tone values recorded during the first stage of labor in the group with oxytocin and the control group without oxytocin, a total recording time of about 250 hours. Abnormal basal tone values are observed in 3% of the control group and in about 10% of the oxytocin group. A similar relationship was found for all other recorded parameters of uterine activity and also for the second stage of labor. Figure 3 shows uterine activity (frequency x intensity of contractions in a period of 10 minutes) in Montevideo units for both groups. Again abnormal uterine activity is about 3 times more frequent in the oxytocin group. It can be concluded therefore, that abnormal uterine activity is found in a small

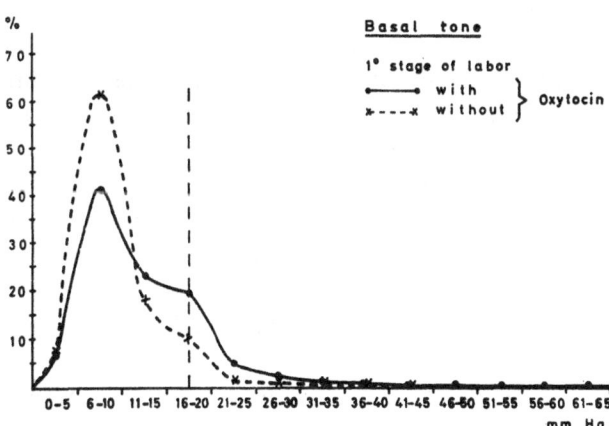

Fig. 2. Frequency distribution of basal tone values during the first stage of labor with and without oxytocin. Total recording time 160 hours. The presumed upper limit of normal basal tone values during the first stage (18 mm Hg) is indicated by a broken line.

In the oxytocin group occasional basal tone values are found up to 65 mm Hg.

percentage (as a rule less than 5%) of spontaneous contractions, and that with oxytocin there is a 2 to 4 fold increased incidence of hyperactive uterine abnormalities.

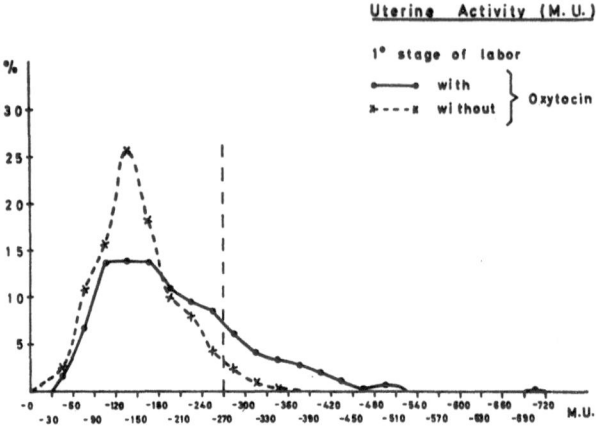

Fig. 3. Frequency distribution of uterine activity in Montevideo units during the first stage of labor with and without oxytocin.
Total recording time 160 hours.
The presumed upper limit of normal uterine activity during the first stage (270 M.U.) is indicated by a broken line.

bb. *Uterine hyperactivity as defined by the cardiovascular reaction of the individual fetus:* It was felt that the definition of abnormal labor on a purely statistical basis was not absolutely satisfactory. Therefore a second approach to the problem was attempted in so far, that abnormal uterine activity was defined not only on the basis of intrauterine pressure data, but also of the individual fetal heart rate response. Abnormal (hyperactive) uterine activity was then defined as an episode of labor where the occurrence of intrauterine pressure values exceeding the average range was accompanied by pathologic fetal heart rate patterns. Examples are given in figures 7 and 8, where uterine hyperactivity causes undefined severe fetal FHR decelerations with reactive tachycardia. Figure 4 demonstrates mild uterine hyperactivity giving rise to a mild late deceleration pattern of FHR.

   The relative incidence of episodes of abnormal uterine activity as defined in this way is given in table 2. They were found in almost 50% of the oxytocin group and 17% of the control group. In an individual patient they occurred more often in the oxytocin group than in the control group. Finally the total time duration of abnormal labor in the oxytocin group was 4 times that in the control group.

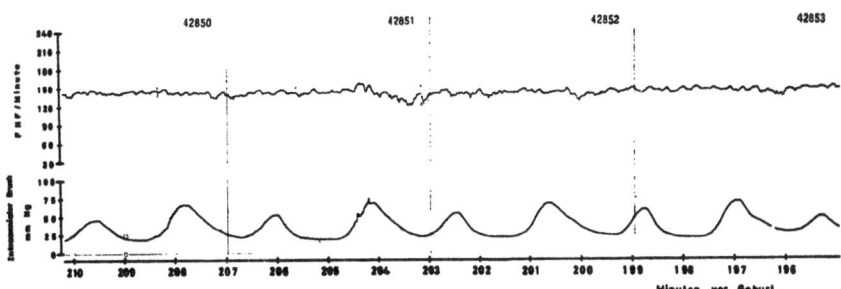

Fig. 4. Uterine hyperactivity (increased basal tone and frequency) resulting in a mild late deceleration pattern of FHR.

Table 2. Incidence of abnormal uterine activity (with abnormal FHR-patterns) with and without oxytocin. Total number of patients with oxytocin 75, without 85.

	with	without
	oxytocin	
Number of patients	36 = 49%	15 = 17,6%
Total number of episodes	60	17
Number of episodes per patient	1,6	1.1
Duration	775 min	184 min
in % of total time of monitoring	7,76%	1,91%

Again it can be concluded that pathologic uterine activity is about 2 to 4 times more frequent with oxytocin stimulation.

c. *Effect of abnormal uterine activity on fetal pH*

Figure 5 gives a more detailed analysis of the pH-difference in umbilical artery blood between the oxytocin group and the control patients. Whereas mean fetal pH is significantly lower in the oxytocin group as a whole, those cases of the oxytocin stimulated group that did not show abnormal uterine activity exhibited a mean fetal pH which was similar to this of the control group. However, fetal pH-values from patients with episodes of abnormal uterine activity were far below the mean pH of either group and this provides strong evidence that abnormal uterine activity accounts at least in part for the difference in mean fetal pH observed between the control group and the oxytocin stimulated group.

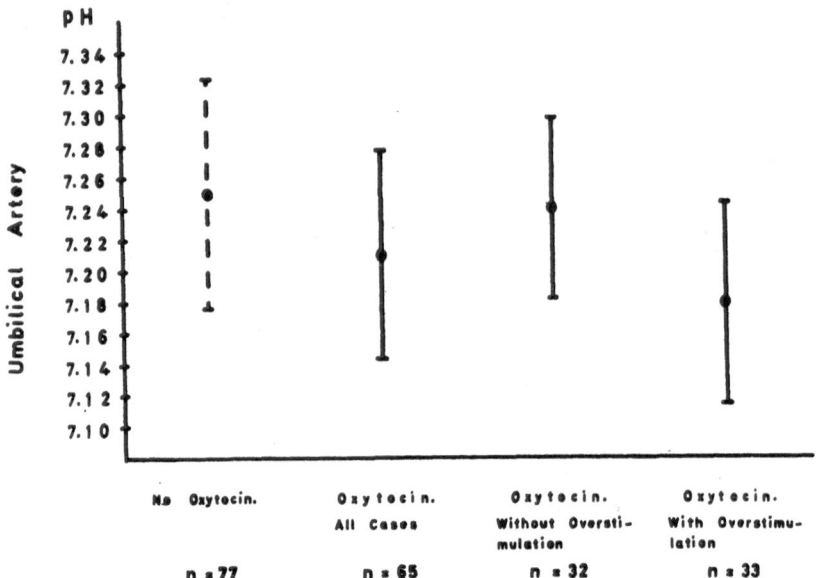

Fig. 5. Analysis of the umbilical artery pH difference between patients with and without oxytocin. When the oxytocin group is divided into sub-groups with and without uterine hyperactivity (overstimulation), the difference to the control group is statistically significant for the subgroup with overstimulation only.

Discussions and conclusions

It is a rather interesting observation that uterine hyperactivity does occur in 17% of spontaneous and apparently uncomplicated labors. More pertinent to the present topic, however, are the findings that abnormal uterine activity is 2 to 4 times more frequent with oxytocin stimulation than with spontaneous labor, furthermore that uterine hyperactivity is accompanied by a significant trend to low fetal pH-values.

This does not mean that oxytocin is a useless drug which should be avoided. But these data point to a inherent risk in the administration of oxytocin. It seems evident that in our practice oxytocin was not administered carefully enough. Adverse effects of oxytocin basically are bound to incorrect dosage, and the problems of oxytocin application are primarily problems of dosage. It is demonstrated in figure 6 that clearcut overdosage of oxytocin was rare in our patients. However two factors may be responsable for some of the shortcomings: 1) With an intravenous infusion the number of drops/minute are not always constant and spontaneous changes in the infusion rate may occur. This situation is demon-

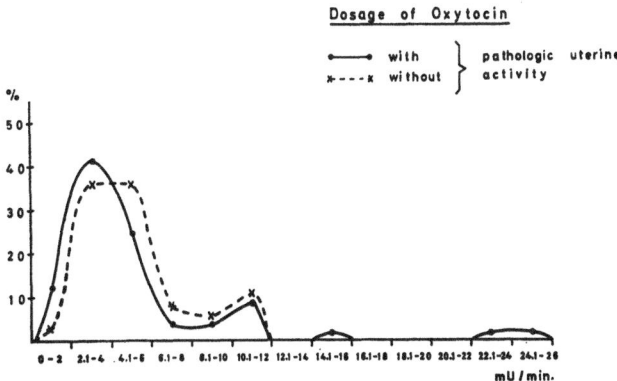

Fig. 6. Frequency distribution of the dosages of oxytocin in patients with and without uterine hyperactivity.

strated in figure 7, showing uterine overstimulation definitly caused by a short period of uncontrolled intravenous infusion. On the other hand individual differences in uterine sensitivity evidently do exist. In figure 8 an example of this type is given: Several attempts of stimulating the uterus by about 3 milliunits of oxytocin/minute were inevitably followed by uterine hyperactivity.

In view of this facts we have decided to administer oxytocin only by infusion-pump, where a constant infusion rate is guaranteed and where very small dosages may be infused. The safest way to give oxytocin is undoubtedly by infusion-pump with simultaneous intrauterine pressure recording. Then following limits should not be exceeded during the first stage: frequency of contractions should not exceed 5 per 10 minutes, intensity should not exceed 60 mm Hg and basal tone should not exceed 15 mm Hg.

In fact, in a more recent series of 75 patients where oxytocin had been given by infusion-pump, periods of uterine hyperactivity were observed in 15 patients or about 20% only.

II. EFFECT OF PARACERVICAL ANESTHESIA ON UTERINE ACTIVITY AND ON THE FETUS

Paracervical anesthesia is a convenient type of anesthesia which is highly estimated by most patients. In recent years, however, some adverse effects of this type of anesthesia on the fetus have been detected and in several studies by Teramo (9), Gordon (10), Jung et al. (11) and others the oc-

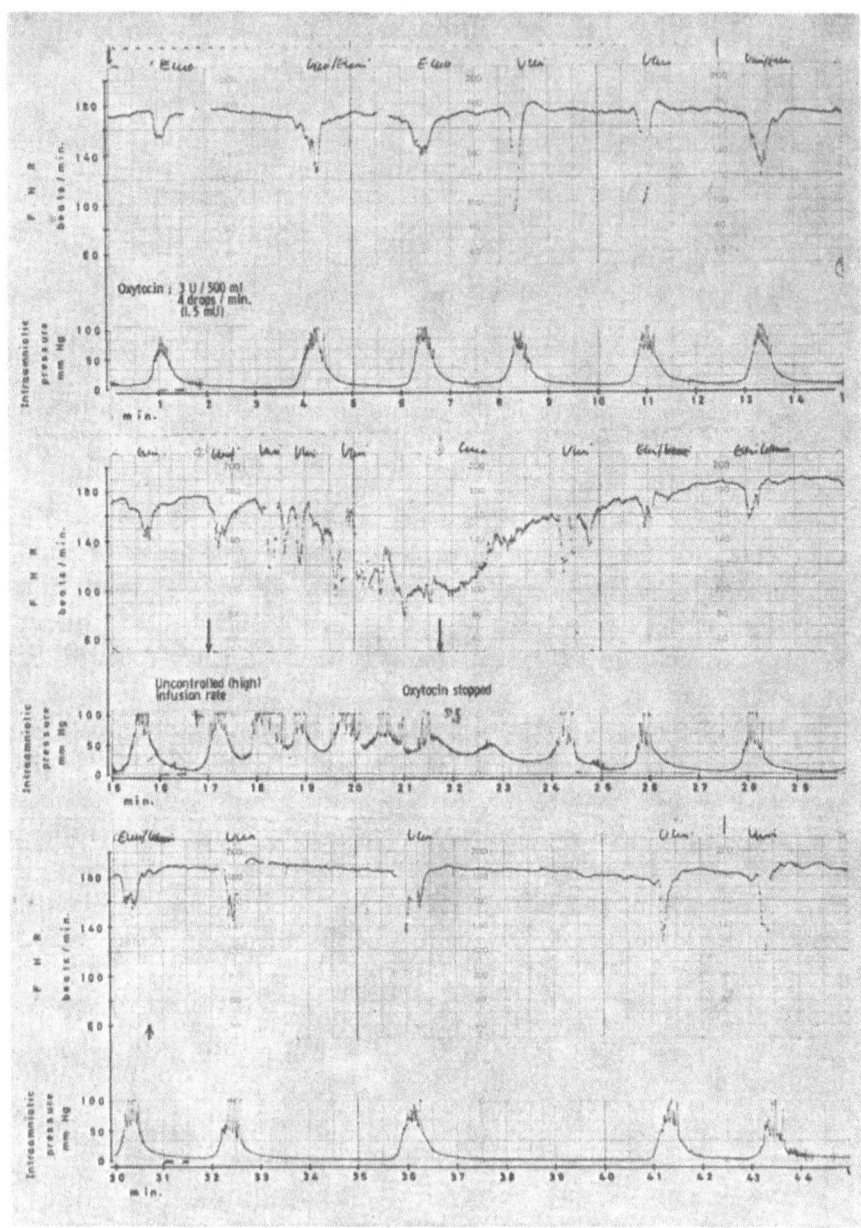

Fig. 7. FHR and intrauterine pressure in a patient with transient and accidental overdosage of oxytocin. Severe undefined FHR deceleration and reactive fetal tachycardia.

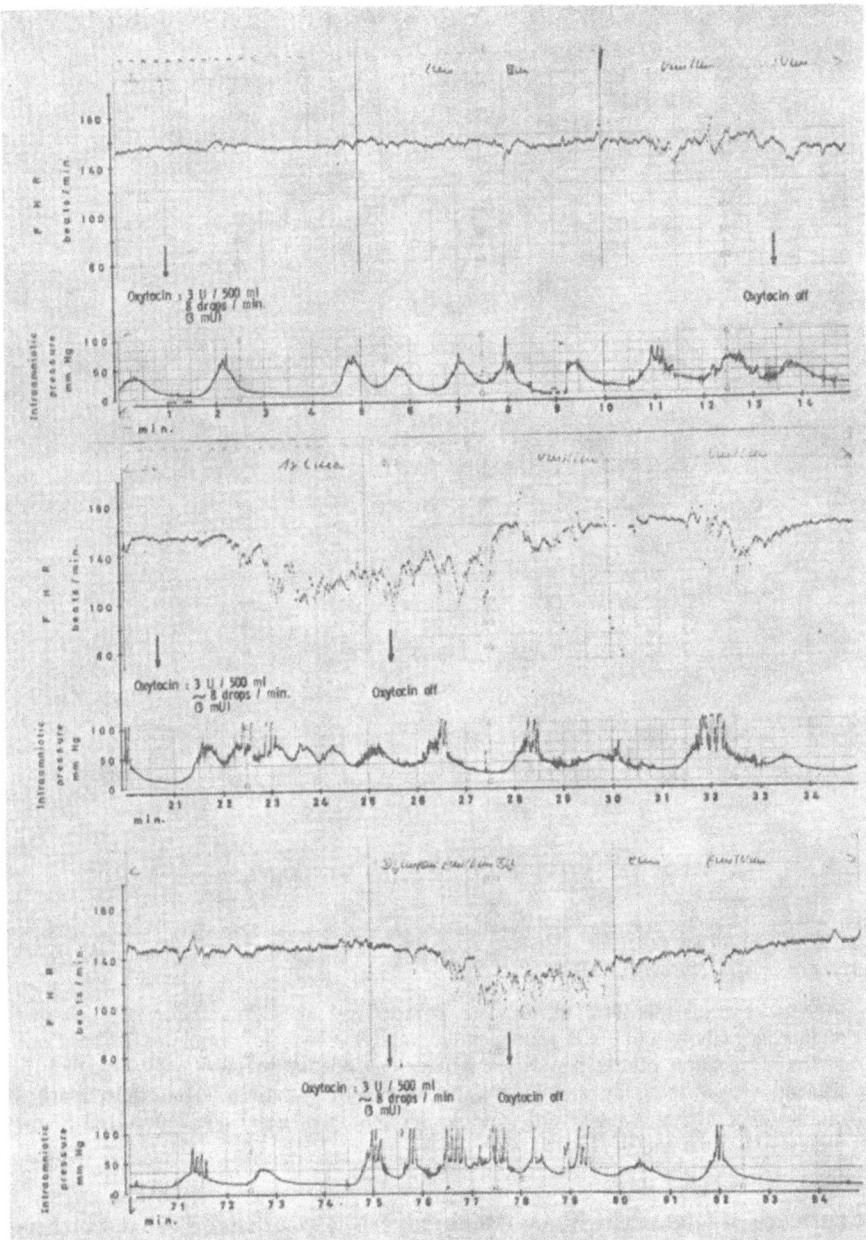

Fig. 8. FHR and intrauterine pressure in a patient with a 'sensitive uterus'. Several attemps of stimulating labor with 3 milliunits of oxytocin result in uterine hyperactivity.

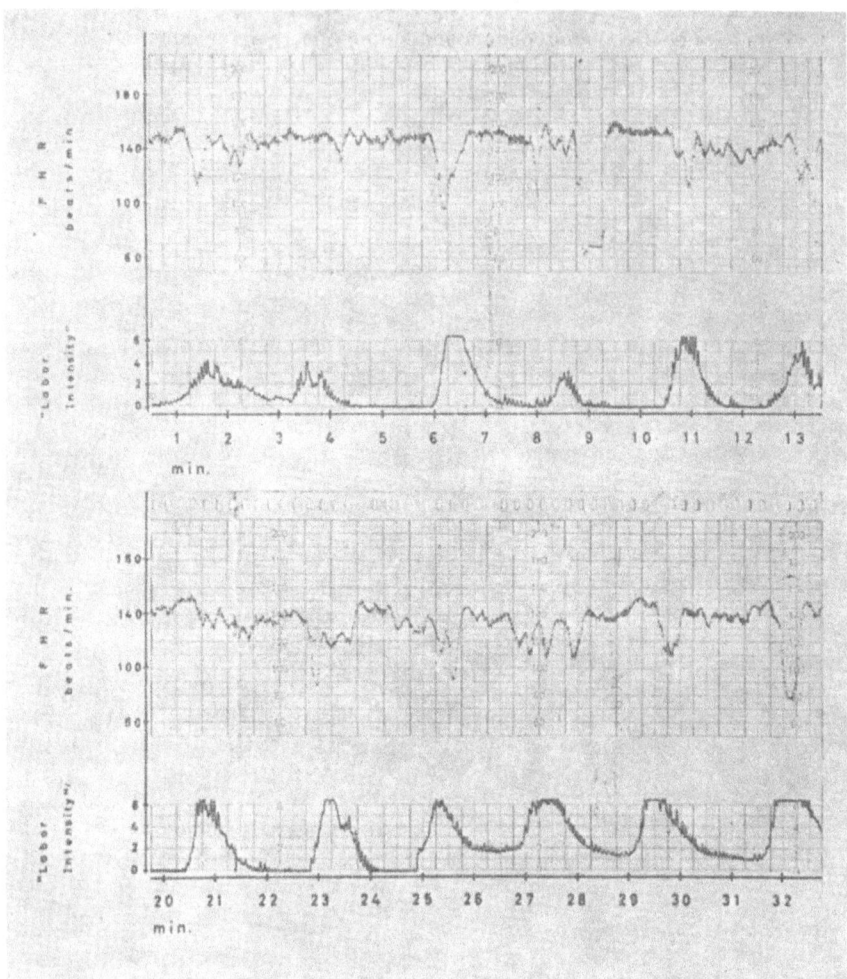

Fig. 9a. Intrapartum fetal death with paracervical anesthesia. External recording of uterine activity and FHR (phonocardiography). Oxytocin stimulated labor. Prior to the application of the paracervical block a tendency to uterine hyperactivity is present, accompanied by a mild variable deceleration pattern. After PCA marked uterine hyperactivity and severe variable decelerations. Fetal death occurred a few minutes after the end of this record.

currence of fetal acidosis and fetal bradycardia was demonstrated. Furthermore some cases of fetal death have been described.

In our department the only intrapartum fetal death in 1968 occurred with paracervical anesthesia. The course of events in this case is demon-

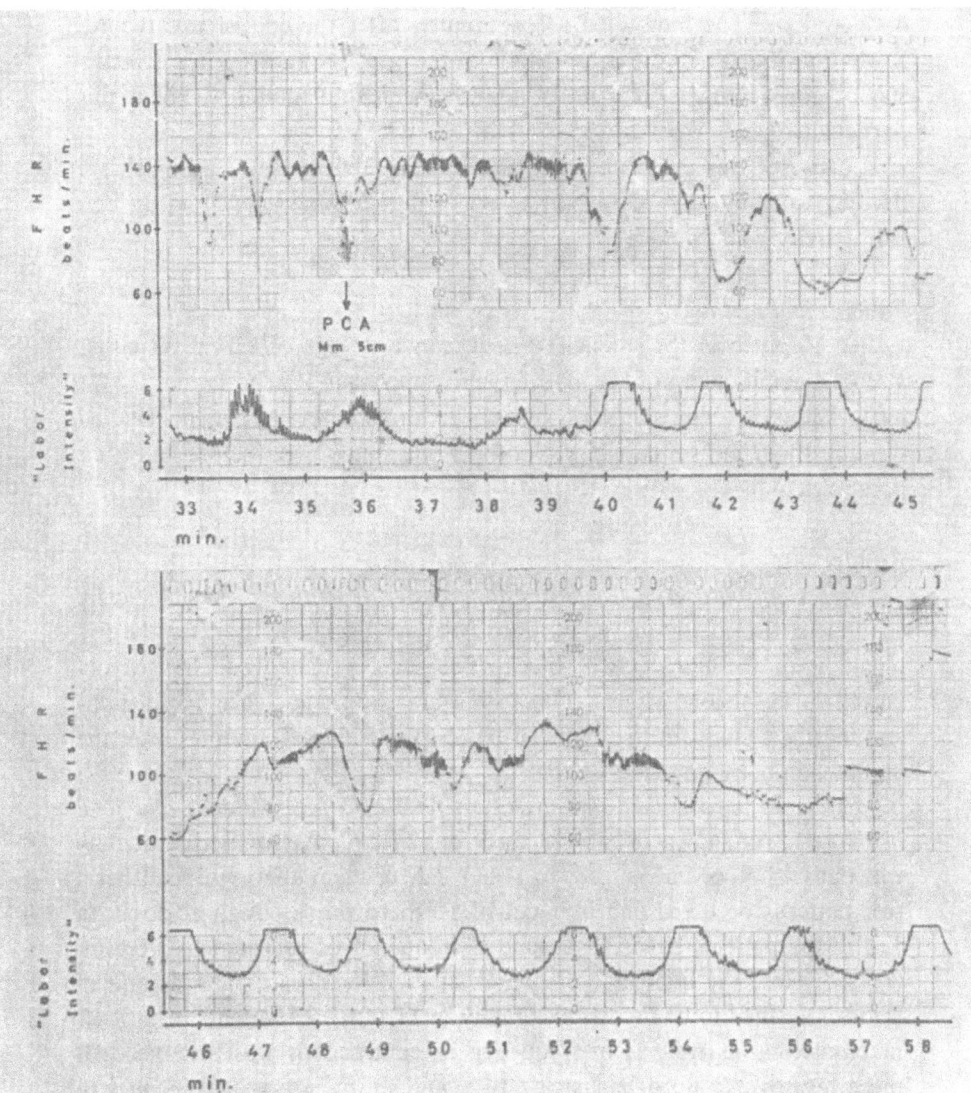

Fig. 9b. See legend fig. 9a.

strated in fig. 9. Paracervical anesthesia was performed in a patient, where the fetus was subject to mild cord compression and where a tendency to uterine hyperactivity with oxytocin stimulation was present. The cord compression pattern increased with increasing uterine activity and after paracervical anesthesia uterine hypertonus occurred with severe variable decelerations. The fetus died a few minutes after the end of this record. It was concluded that the combination of the effect of paracervical anesthesia, of cord compression and of uterine overstimulation had killed this particular fetus.

Because of this event and of observations published by Jung (11), we decided to study more closly the effect of paracervical anesthesia on uterine activity.

Patients and methods
Either Mepivacain (Scandicain) 1% in single dosage of 12 ml on either side or a combination of Mepivacain and Bupivacain (Carbostesine) 0.5%, again 12 ml on either side were given. The total number of patients studied was 35. In 27 fetuses capillary blood pH was determined before and after paracervical block.

Results
a. *Effect of paracervical anesthesia on uterine activity:* A statistically significant rise in uterine activity was observed immediatly after the application of the paracervical block. The most pronounced changes occurred in basal tone values. These data are shown in figure 10, demonstrating the significant rise in mean basal tone within 10 minutes after the application of the paracervical block.
b. *Effect of paracervical anesthesia on fetal acid base balance and fetal heart rate:* As shown in table 3, in 9 out of 27 patients uterine activity was diminished or unchanged. In about half of them abnormal fetal heart rate patterns occurred and in 1 out of 10 there was a definit acidosis. In 1/4 of the patients either basal tone of frequency of contractions were increased. Here the incidence of abnormal fetal heart rate patterns and of acidosis seemed to be increased. Finally in 11 of the 27 patients an increase in basal tone as well as in frequency of contractions was observed. Of these fetuses one third had an acidosis and the majority had changes in fetal heart rate patterns and pH.

Discussion
The mechanism by which paracervical anesthesia exerts its adverse effect on the fetus is not known. Several hypothesis have been brought forward. We have been inclined to believe that direct myocardial depression by the local anesthetic is a major factor. But on the basis of the data shown we

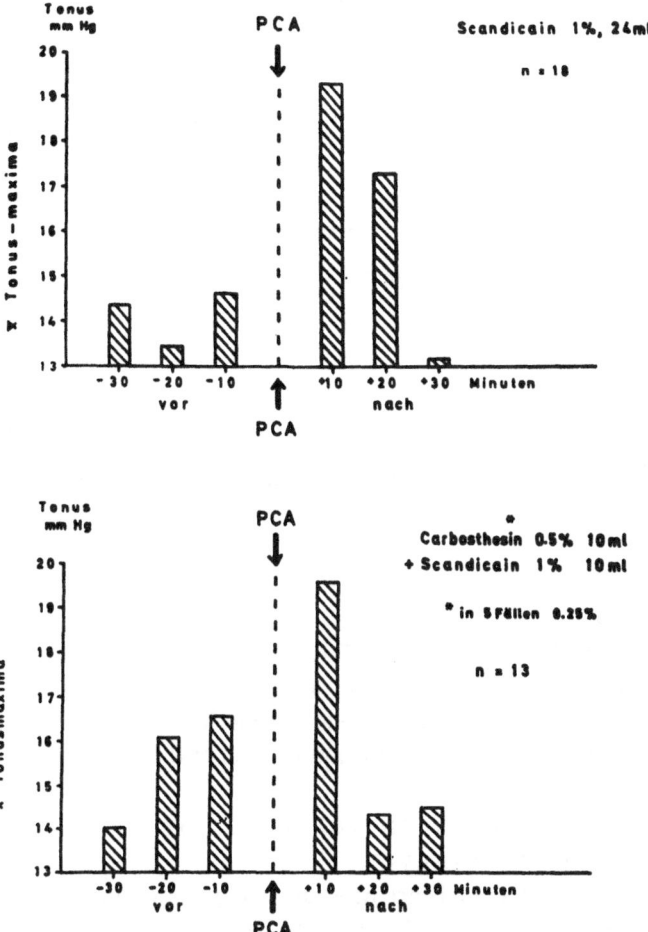

Fig. 10. Basal tone values before and after paracervical block with two different drugs.
The differences before and after paracervical block are significant statistically.

also feel that this is not necessarily the whole story. There is some evidence that uterine activity may be influenced by paracervical anesthesia and that hyperactivity does occur in part of these cases. Evidently fetal asphyxia with paracervical anesthesia is modified and definitly enhanced by the occurrence of uterine hyperactivity. For practical purposes the combination of paracervical anesthesia and oxytocin application seems to be especially dangerous. On a theoretical level the observations of De Mot et al. (12) suggesting that both, uterine hyperactivity and fetal acidosis

Table 3. Changes of FHR and fetal acid base balance with PCA in relationship to associated changes of uterine activity.

Uterine Activity	n	Abnormal FHR-Patterns	Decrease in pH > 0.03	Fetal Acidosis pH < 7.25
Decrease or unchanged	9 (33%)	5 (55%)	2 (22%)	1 (11%)
Increase of Frequency only	5 (26%)	2	3	1
Increase of Basal Tone only	2	1	–	–
Increase of Basal Tone and Frequency	11 (41%)	9 (82%)	9 (82%)	4 (36%)
Total	27 (100%)	17 (63%)	15 (55%)	6 (22%)

might be the consequence of uterine ischemia induced by the paracervical block, are of special interest.

We are still performing paracervical anesthesia. However a very strict selection is done, and paracervical anesthesia is applied in the presence of normal fetal acid base balance and normal fetal heart rate only, and no oxytocin is given at the time of the application of the anesthesia.

III. ADVERSE EFFECT ON THE FETUS OF THE MONITORING PROCEDURES THEMSELVES

The monitoring of fetal heart rate and contractions in our opinion is a most useful tool in modern obstetrics. In closing this paper we would draw attention to the possibility that adverse effects may be bound also to this procedure.

One of these adverse effects is the occurrence of a maternal supine hypotensive syndrom when monitoring is done by phonocardiography. The most favorable maternal position for this type of monitoring is the supine position. This in turn, however, may be the cause of fetal compromise resulting in pathologic fetal records. Figure 11 may give an example: severe maternal hypotension during monitoring was observed at several occasions in a twin pregnancy. In figure 11 the fetal cardiovascular reaction to this event is shown: Severe deceleration of fetal heart rate with reactive tachycardia and loss of beat-to-beat fluctuation. In this patient maternal hypotension was easily recognised as cause of fetal hypoxia. But we also

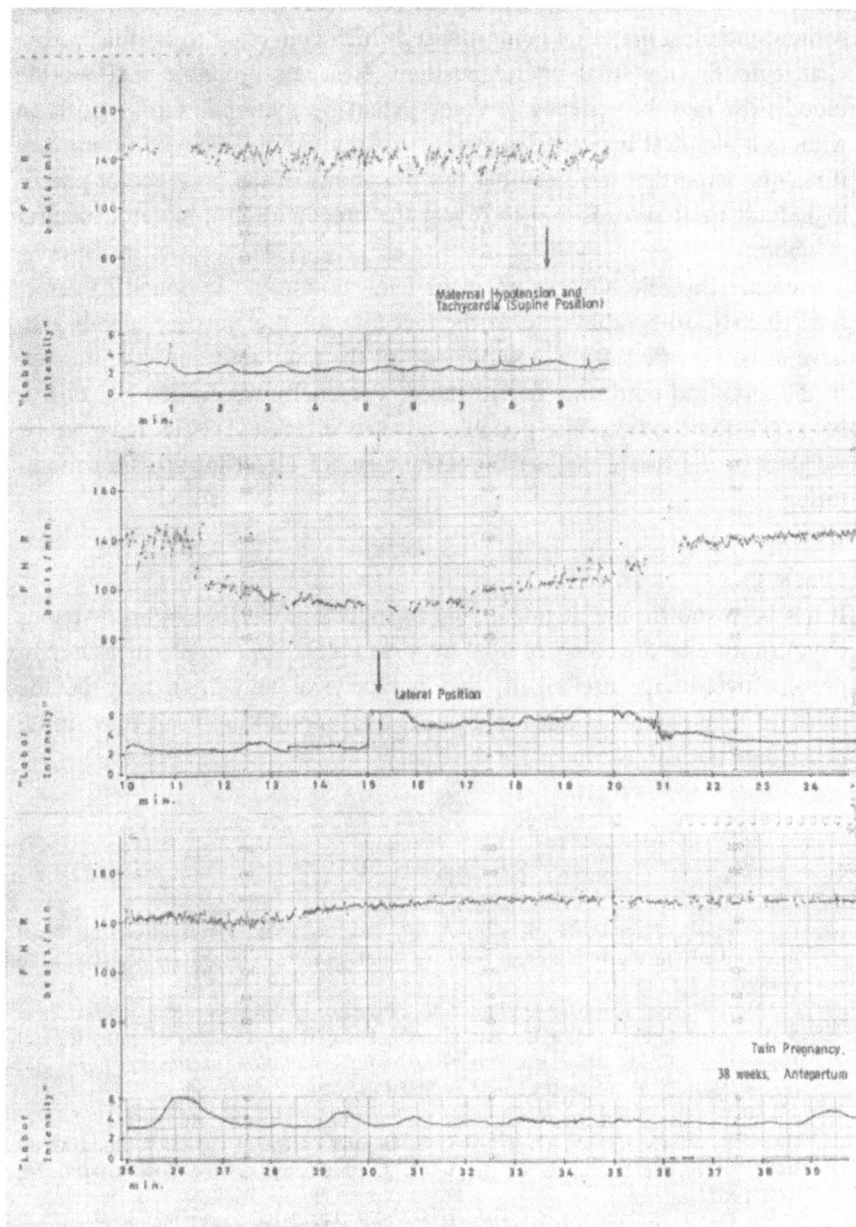

Fig. 11. Severe maternal hypotension during external FHR-monitoring by phono-cardiography in a supine position. Undefined FHR deceleration, reactive loss of beat-to-beat fluctuation and tachycardia.

observed, in maternal supine position, consistent pathologic fetal records without manifest maternal compromise, which converted to normal with a change to the maternal lateral position. It seems probable that uterine blood flow may be reduced to some extent by maternal supine position without a manifest hypotensive syndrow. Although this may be rather rare it may be important to remember this possibility in the presence of pathologic fetal FHR records and to repeat the procedure in a maternal lateral position.

Another possible adverse effect of fetal monitoring is bound to direct fetal electrocardiography and to the fact that for this purpose membranes have to be ruptured. Both, compression of the fetal head and compression of the umbilical cord may be enhanced. Personally we do not feel this to be a substantial risk, but possible adverse effect (11) will have to be weighed in the future against the advantages of direct intrapartum monitoring.

SUMMARY

It has been shown that augmentation or induction of labor by intravenous oxytocin may be the cause of fetal hypoxia unless appropriate measures to prevent overdosage are taken; that paracervical anesthesia may be the cause of fetal asphyxia, and finally that fetal monitoring itself may, in an occasional patient, compromise the fetus.

REFERENCES

1. Kubli F. W., Hon E. H., Khazin A. F., Takemura H., Observations on heart rate and pH in the human fetus during labor. *Amer. J. Obst. Gynec.* 104, 1190 (1969).
2. Caldeyro-Barcia R., Mendez-Bauer C., Poseiro J. J., Escarcena L. A., Pose S. V., Arnt I. C., Gullin L., Althabe O., Bieniarz J., Control of human fetal heart rate during labor. In: *The heart and circulation in the newborn and infant.* (Ed. D. E. Cassel) Grune & Stratton, New York 1966.
3. Saling E., *Das Kind im Bereich der Geburtshilfe.* Thieme, Stuttgart 1966.
4. Beard R. W., Morris E. D., Clayton S. G., pH of foetal capillary blood as an indicator of the condition of the fetus. *J. of Obstet. Gynec. Brit. Cwlth.* 74, 812, 1967.
5. Kubli F. W., *Foetale Gefahrenzustände und ihre Diagnose.* Thieme, Stuttgart, 1966.
6. Caldeyro-Barcia R., Poseiro J. J., Physiology of the uterine contractions. *Clin. Obstet. Gynec.* 3, 386, 1969.
7. Cibils L. A., Hendricks Ch., Normal labor in vertex presentation. *Amer. J. Obstet. & Gynec.* 91, 385 (1965).

8. Caldeyro-Barcia, R., Kraphol A. J., Uterine contractions in spontaneous labor. *Amer. J. Obstet. Gynec.* 106, 378 (1970).
9. Teramo K., Studies on foetal acid-base values after paracervical blockade during labor. *Acta Obstet. Gynec.* 48, 80 (1969).
10. Gordon H. R., Fetal bradycardia after paracervical block. *New Engl. J. Med.* 279, 910 (1968).
11. Jung H., Dopecky P., Klöck F. K., Zur fetalen Gefährdung bei der Paracervical-blockade. *Gebh. Frauenhlk.* 30, 463, (1970).
12. Mot de E. et al., Le risque foetal dans l'anésthésie paracervicale: rôle joué par l'hypertonie utérine. *Proceedings of the 2nd European Congress of Perinatal Medicine,* London 1970. In press.
13. Schwarcz R. L., Strada-Saenz, G., Althabe, O., Fernandez-Funes, J., Caldeyro-Barcia, R., Pressure exerted by uterine contractions on the head of the human fetus during labor. In: *Perinatal factors affecting human development.* Proceedings of the special session held during the 8th Meeting of the *PAHO* Advisory Committee on Medical Research 10 June 1969 in Washington, D.C. Scientific publication No. 185.

THE INFLUENCE OF ANAESTHETIC DRUGS ON THE FOETUS AND NEWBORN

D. T. POPESCU

Although as early as 1858 Spaeth mentioned the first drug passing the placenta (potassium iodine in syphilis treatment) (1) we used, for years and years, to consider placenta as a strong barrier between mother and foetus.

Much progress was done in the last 10 years: improved laboratory techniques allowed a better knowledge of the anatomy, physiology and pathology of the placenta, we got a better comprehension of physico-chemical laws governing the passage of drugs across it and thus of the influence of various drugs on the foetus and newborn. The theories of the respiratory uptake and elimination of inhalational anaesthetics, the theories of dynamic distribution of intravenous administered drugs, the better understanding of drug metabolism and elimination brought anaesthetic theory on a higher level and allowed it to be fruitfully applied in obstetrics. The biochemical research on enzymes in mother and child, represent another step further in comprehension of drug action on the newborn. Much was written on these subjects, experimental works, clinical observations or clinical studies. But we have to be careful in interpreting the data from literature because on one side it is demonstrated that anatomically and physiologically placentas are different in various mammalian species, on the other side clinical cases are important – but isolated – cases and sometimes wrongly interpreted (2) while clinical trials are difficult because ethical conditions, the delicate laboratory techniques and the imponderable of anaesthesiologists own skill. Even so we must recognise that much of what is known, has been learnt on man, for therapeutic necessity has produced many inpromptu human experiments in this field (3).

At present a step was reached when we can say that placenta is no more a barrier but a living tissue between mother and foetus, that the effect of the drugs used in anaesthesia is almost the same in the foetus and newborn as in the mother and that the most important problem is not which drug is passing through the placenta but how much from a certain drug reaches the foetus, the rate and mechanism of transfer involved (4).

It is impossible for me in the time allowed, to enumerate all the drugs passing the placenta with rates, coefficients, quantities and their influence on the newborn. It is also valueless to you to listen to a pure enumeration of data. I therefore prefer to point out the understanding of our problem.

Three phenomena are to be considered in this regard:

– the distribution of drugs in the organism of the mother
– the mechanisms of placental transfer
– the particularities of foetal anatomy and physiology explaining the different effect of various drugs.

I. DISTRIBUTION OF DRUGS

Distribution of drugs in the mothers organism in most important, because the first condition for a drug influencing the foetus is its presence in the mothers circulation.

For inhalation anaesthetics the blood concentration is dependent on:

– concentration offered
– ventilatory conditions of the mother
– air/blood and blood/lipid partition coefficients and solubility
– circulatory condition of the mother.

All these problems governing inhalational anaesthesia are well known to anaesthetists.

For injected drugs Paton (5) suggested, that, subsequent to the intravenous injection of a concentrated solution, the drug is travelled like a bolus, or 'slug' for two or three complete circulations before beeing equally diffused throughout the blood. Price (6) showed that distribution of Pentothal is based on the perfusion debit of organs. The first to get a high amount of a drug injected intravenously in a concentrated form, will be the best irrigated organs: brain, heart, viscera, placenta, while lean body mass (skin, muscles) start the uptake only 15 minutes later and fat (poorly irrigated) some 1 hour later (fig. 1).

Therefore, the haemodynamic balance of the patient is of paramount importance in barbiturate induction:

– a haemorrhagic person (frequently in obstetrics) with low cardiac minutevolume (shunts open) will get a very quick and high concentration of drug in the brain – but also in uterus and placenta – and thus in the foetal circulation.

– a hypermetabolic, hyperthyreoidean or simply anxious agitated patient with an extremely quick circulation time and well irrigated lean body mass will necessitate high doses for the saturation of lean tissue which will take up rapidly the circulating drug minimising thus the brain concentration (fig. 2).

Selwyn-Crawford and Rudofski (7) made subsequent calculations based on the above mentioned theories and considered also the obstetric consequences. They speculated on the mode of injecting 250 mg Pentothal: in concentrated form (in 9 seconds), in dilute form (in 5 minutes), in very dilute form-infusion-(in 25 minutes) (fig. 3).

We can see that in the first case (concentrated dose) the maximal

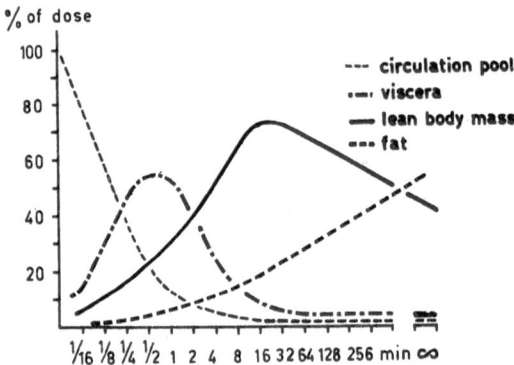

Fig. 1. % concentration of dose.

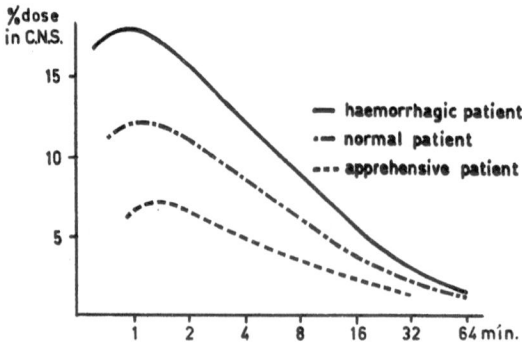

Fig. 2. Influence of circulation.

effective dose will be attained in the central nervous system in 30 seconds
while in the very dilute form (infusion in 25 minutes) (fig. 3) an utile
concentration will be obtained only after the completion of the infusion
(after some 27 minutes).

At the same time the plasma concentration will fall rapidly in the first
two cases (fig. 4), while in the last one a high plasma level will be obtained
between 18 and 30 minutes after the start of the infusion.

The implications for the foetus are that high umbilical blood levels will
be obtained after some 8 minutes in the rapid injection technique (a plea
for the rapid method in caesarean section) (fig. 5), while the same concen-

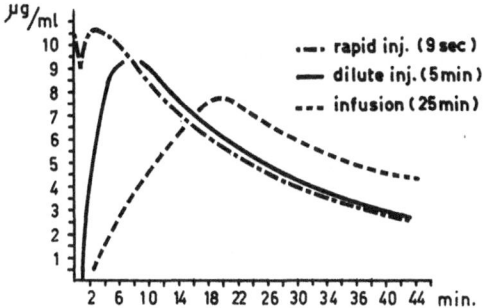

Fig. 3. Concentration in CNS.

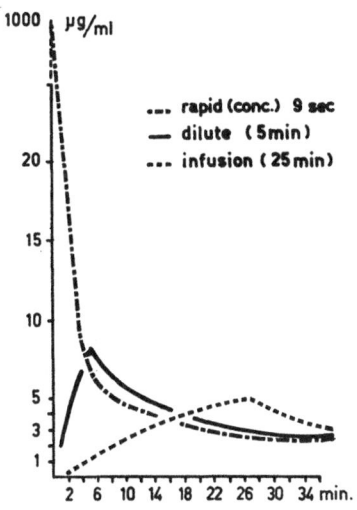

Fig. 4. Concentration in blood ug/ml.

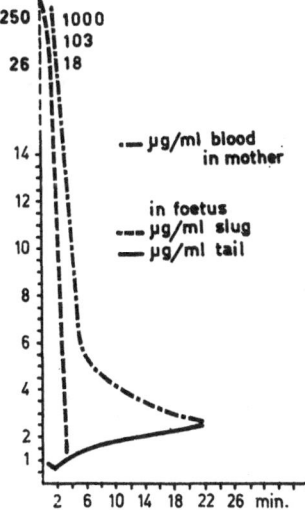

Fig. 5. Concentration injection.

trations in foetal blood will be obtained but in some 12 minutes by the dilute injection (fig. 6), and in some 22 minutes in the infusion technique (fig. 7).

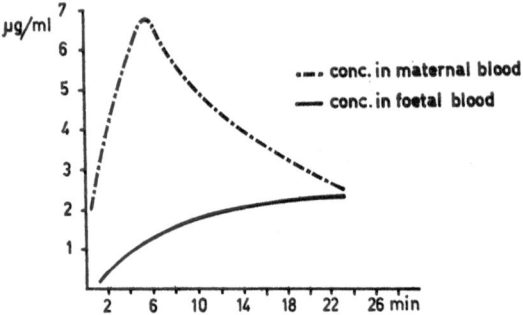

Fig. 6.　Diluted inj. (5 min.).

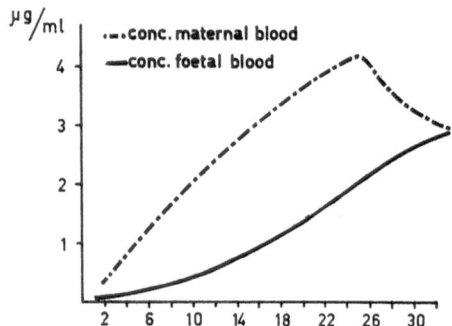

Fig. 7.　Very dilute inj. (infusion).

An intramuscularly injected drug will be absorbed slowly into circulation giving a curve resembling to the perfusion technique. In this case the metabolic inactivating factors, as well as excretion processes, have time enough to play a role in the final amount of drug offered to placental transfer (table 1). The graphic reproduced here belongs to a former work of Selwyn Crawford (8). Three times more promazine was found in the neonates after 50 mg of this drug injected intravenously to their mothers as when the same quantity was administered by intramuscular way. When the drug was administered by intravenous infusion, the quantity was nearly 4 times, for in prolonged administration, time plays an important role in transfer.

The work of Selwyn-Crawford on the transmission of Pethidine (9) as

Table 1.

50 mg Promazine to mother	Elimination Promazine in neonatal urine	
	Max. concentration	Total / 48 h
I. Musc.	0,063	9,2
I. Ven	0,303	28,2
Perfusion	0,250	34,0

the recent work of Thomas (10) of the placental transfer of Alcuronium also support this point of view.

II. TRANSFER THROUGH THE PLACENTA

Anatomically constructed as a sandwich of fibrinoid tissue – Nitabuch's layer – with double origin: maternal and embrionic, between two layers of cells – the deciduals – maternal in origin and the trophoblast from embrionic origin, placenta represents a peculiar organ offering the foetus the priviliged situation of homograft (11) being in the same time: lung, kidney, intestine, liver and endocrine gland.

The transfer of molecules through it is correlated with maternal and foetal blood flow. This represents a serious difficulty in prediction of passage of drugs because even in normal child birth blood flow in the uterus and the foetal exocorporeal circulation are many times considerably altered in an unknown degree (12). In parturients at term placental blood flow is 600–750 ml/min (13), but diminishes significantly during long and sustained contractions. When intra uterine pressure exceeds 40 mm Hg (normal pressure in ombilical vein) (14) the placental circulation stops and thus the passage of gasses or soluble molecules. The position of the mother can modify placental passage by circulatory changes brought by the compressing uterus.

The problem is even more complicated by the lobar pattern of placental circulation, different lobes having nearly always different blood flow rates (1).

Anyhow hypotension in mother is one of the most dangerous incidents for the foetus and hypocapnia, through maternal vasoconstriction, produces foetal anoxia (and acidosis but this will be dealed on later). Other pathologic factors as anoxia, dehydration, preeclampsia, erythroblastosis, diabetes mellitus, infarction of placental lobes and so on will modify the normal passage also. It is even difficult to ascertain what 'normal' means, because we sometimes see the so called 'placental barrier' completely breaking down as it is shown by foetal red cells in the maternal circulation (3) without pathological significance. Since long it was demonstrated that small molecules (mol. weigth less than 600) pass easily while those over 1000 slowly. This generated the theory of

1. *Ultrafiltration* (table 2). Fifty years ago placenta was regarded as a simple semipermeable membrane similar to endothelial walls of blood vessels. Barcroft and others seriously questioned this mechanism.

Table 2. Mechanisms of placental transfer

Usual processes

Ultrafiltration

Diffusion $\Big\langle$ simple / facilitated

Rate of diffusion $= k \; \dfrac{Area \; (Cmat–Cfoet)}{Thickness}$

Active transport $\Big\langle$ unmodified / inactivated

Special processes
Pinocytosis
Breaks in villi

---

2. *Diffusion* is the second mechanism described whether it is *simple* or *facilitated*. Simple diffusion is based on Fick's law, the factors being; the gradient of concentrations in maternal and foetal blood, the area of contact, the time of contact (influenced by blood flow on both sides), the thickness of the membrane, and a diffusion constant particular to every drug. It must be emphasized that for a rapid diffusion the drug must have a high lipid solubility and a low degree of ionisation.

Facilitated diffusion is explained by carrier molecules oscillating rapidly between the two interfaces of the placental membrane. It is necessary to admit this mechanism, for equilibrium is achieved for many substances more rapidly than would be predicted on physico-chemical grounds alone. But we must keep in mind that placenta is a living organ having its own metabolism, consuming oxygen, producing carbon dioxyde and other

metabolites and containing a big number of enzymes. These are responsible for:

3. *Active transport mechanism,* various molecules are temporary combined to membrane enzyme systems. Metabolic energy will be consumed
for this sort of transport required to pass certain ions, big molecules or
foreign compounds.

4. *Special processes are: Pinocitosis* – droplets of plasma engulfed by
microscopic invaginations of the villi of placental cells and,

Breaks in the placenta villi explaining transfer of whole cells. The last
mechanisms are probably not important for drug transfer. Any combination of the above mentioned mechanisms are possible at a certain moment
(4). Anaesthetic gases and volatiles pass easily (most of them having also
a high lipid solubility). Barbiturates have also no difficulty to find their
way through the placenta. The same being true for analgesics. Because
of their bigger molecule, high ionisation and low fat solubility, competitive
muscle relaxants (exception gallamine) pass very slowly. It was said that
small doses (till 30 mg tubarine) do not pass. Thomas et al. (10) demonstrated that total dose has little importance, the quantity of Alcuronium
found in the neonates blood is high in case of slow injection to the mother
and low or nul by rapid injection. This correlates with circulatory data
proposed by Paton (25), rapid administration being correlated with rapid
uptake by neuromuscular endplates while slow injection creates a smaller
concentration, but the time contact with placenta is in this case sufficient
to allow passage of the drug. However big doses pass in a high proportion
and Older and Harris (15) quote an apnoeic child resuscitated by edro-
phonium-neostigmine, born by a mother whose status epilepticus was
treated by intubation and intermitent positive pressure ventilation for some
days (a total of 245 mg d Tubocurarine).

Recent studies demonstrated that the rich enzymatic equipment of placenta is able to interfere with drug transmission in the sense of inactivating
some compounds. *Enzymatic modifications.* In regard 'suxamethonium
impermeability of placenta' we know that the drug passes easily but the
high levels of cholin-esterase in placenta inactivate the drug immediately.
The same enzyme is inactivating Propanidid, Procaine and Tetracaine,
which have thus no demonstrable effect on the child (16) while the non
hydrolysable local anaesthetics (Mepivacaine, Lidocaine, Prilocaine) being
liposoluble and having a low ionisation rate pass easily, are not enzyma-
tically modified and can depress the child.

The high level of mono-aminoxydase is inactivating epinephrine which, although passing rapidly, has no direct effect on the foetus. Placental enzymatic activity is also responsible for the inactivation of serotonine and histamine. It is interesting to note that addition of epinephrine to local anaesthetics will produce lower maternal and foetal plasmatic levels of anaesthetic, but as local vasoconstriction in mother occurs the abcorption of the drug will be slower, the factor time starts to play an important part and the concentration of drugs will be nearly the same in the child as in mothers plasma (table 3).

Table 3

	Administered dose	Blood concentration	
		in mother	in neonate
Lidocaine 1,5% plain	502 ± 218	2,6 ± 1,3	1,8 ± 0,9
Lidocaine 1,5% + epinephrine	424 ± 169	1,7 ± 0,8	1,6 ± 0,8

We can conclude this problem saying that all the anaesthetic drugs are passing and that placenta, has an active participation in the transmission of molecules, for or against the passage, sometimes metabolising drugs, but it is neither a simply dialising membrane nor an absolute barrier.

III. INFLUENCE ON THE NEONATE

As was pointed out earlier, the particularities of the foetal circulation will explain some differences in action: 7/8 of umbilical blood flow is passing through the liver thus slowing its speed in reaching the target organs, 1/8 is short circuited in vena cava inferior and diluted with blood coming from the lower extremities (14). In its way to brain the fresh placental blood is even more diluted in the right atrium with cephalic and upper extremity blood and so, a much lower concentration of drug, as that found in the umbilical vein, will reach the foetus central nervous system.

But we must remember that blood-brain barrier in foetus is more permeable than in adults and therefore barbiturates (by example) are more toxic to him (12). Hypoxia, hypercapnia and acidosis are decreasing the strength of the blood-brain barrier and render, in this way, barbiturates or local anaesthetics even more toxic to 'pathologic' foetus (17, 18). The relative renal insufficiency has to be stressed (12) in the neonatal period (impossibility to concentrate urine). This renders dangerous all drugs with renal elimination (competitive relaxants) and also enzymatic defficiences associated with foetal and neonatal life (inability to syntethise some proteins, deficiency in co-factors, enzymes with different activity as in the adult, the presence of inhibitors) (12). The younger the foetus, the more imperfect his enzymatic systems and his organs. Therefore prematurity is said to be the greatest hazard to infants (17).

The influence of drugs on the neonate are, as in adults, also conditioned by concomitant use of certain other compounds in the sense of summation, potentiation or antagonism (18).

It must also be stressed that the (physiologic – or pathologic) condition of the foetus has a first hand influence on the drug action. It is very important to remember that a depressed child will badly tolerate even low doses of general (17) or local anaesthetics (19, 20). Doses with no deleterious effect on a healthy, vigorous foetus at term, can be fatal to an anoxyc, acidotic premature.

Considering the action of anaesthetic drugs on the foetus we have also to take into account the developmental moment when they are administered. Older and Harris (15) quote a case when a child with multiple arthrogriphosis was born by a mother who had prolonged curarisation during the third month of pregnancy for tetanus treatment. Experimentally the same abnormality can be produced in animals by curarising the mother in the time when articulations develop in embryo.

In comparing drug action in neonate and adults we are still handicapped by our lack of knowledge. It was demonstrated (21) and generally accepted that neonates are resistant to succinylcholine. A recent work (2) overthrows our earlier convictions, demonstrating that if we scale the dose not on mg/kg body weight but on mg/m² of surface area, we will conclude that neonates have the same sensibility to succinylcholine as the adults but are more sensitive to d-Tubocurarine.

Another drug with 'difference of influence' – trichloroetilene received also a quantitative explanation recently (21). It was observed that Trilene was more depressant for the foetus than for the mother. The reason consists of the fact that Trichloraetilene concentrates in the lipoid membrane of the red cells. The foetus with his physiologic polyglobulaenia will have a higher concentration of drug (in mg/ml blood) and thus will reach a deeper plane of anaesthesia as his mother.

Atropine, just like in adults was demonstrated to have a bifasic action (22): the rapid passage producing tachycardia while slow passage bradycardia alone or, first bradycardia followed by tachycardia.

Over the local anaesthetics I can repeat that those which are hydrolised by plasma cholinesterase (Procaine, Tetracaine) will have no effect on the foetus, although passing the placenta (16) while aminic compounds non hydrolised (Mepivacaine, Lidocaine, Bupivacaine) can have prolonged foetal depressant action (20, 23) in decrescent order of their enumeration depending on their ability to pass the placenta which is in the same direction. Prilocaine can produce methemoglobinaemia in the neonate as in adults (19). Reviewing the literature we can see that the choice of a particular local anaesthetic drug is made, as a matter of fact more on ground of personal experience and preference and is based more on the consistency of analgetic results in the mother than on the influence in the newborn.

Comparing this time regional techniques, and no more drugs, we can say that spinal anaesthesia (24) has the advantage of the small quantity of drug injected (50–75 mg) and thus brings for the foetus only the danger of hypotension. Careful prophylactic rehydration of the mother significantly reduces this danger. Peridural techniques, as well as regional infiltration techniques (para cervical, perineal and so on) are associated, apart the adverse effect of potential hypotension, with the administration of 300–500 mg of anaesthetic drug which passing in high amounts the placenta can endanger the foetus. Addition of epinephrine, frequently used with these techniques, brings the danger of uterine muscle depression (18) or, can decrease uterine blood flow and thus deprime and acidify the foetus (25). But in the first place when we are administering spinal or peridural techniques to parturients we must keep attention to circulatory changes in pregnancy. This means: compression of vena cava inferior by the pregnant uterus which brings important dilatation of peridural veins with consequent reduction of the peridural spreading place for anaesthetics and maybe reduction of cerebro-spinal fluid. Therefore the spinal or peridural doses are to be reduced with some 30% (26, 27, 28) or else dangerous high levels of anaesthesia will be obtained explaining the frequency of accidents formerly associated with these techniques and wrongly attributed to a 'higher sensibility' of parturients for them.

We did not yet make special investigations in Leiden over anaesthesia in obstetrics; our experience and observations are limited on the conditions of newborn after caesarean sections. Our best results were obtained when the chord was clamped between 5 and 8 minutes after the injection of ± 250 mg Pentothal. This correlates well with the data of Selwyn Crawford and Moya and with the comprehension of the mechanism of placental transfer of drugs discussed above. The newborn is less depressed when he is quickly separated from the maternal circulation, because although he has at that moment a higher proportion of barbiturate in his circulation than 10 minutes later, we have to remember that the total amount of drug passed in the foetus and fixed in the C.N.S. is much higher after 12 than after 5 minutes, after the injection of Pentothal to the mother. The results are perhaps less pertinent when we compare the two anaesthetic techniques, after an induction dose of 250 mg than after a 500 mg one.

In the quick technique we are seldom obliged to administer a second dose of succinylcholine (appart the ± 75 mg for intubation) thus we have less risk for the newborn, while for the mother the technique brings no risk of awareness during the operation as does the slow induction operation technique.

We prefer to ventilate the mother with pure oxigen till the chord is clamped.

We can safely administer 0.75% methoxyflurane to the mother immediately after intubation, the concentration is low and brings no further risk to the newborn, but ensures a good analgesia to the mother, permits a 100% oxigenation, a minimal dose of relaxant-post partum, maintains a good uterine contractility and allows the usual dosage of oxytocic drugs.

We agree with Bessem (29) that the participation of a fulltrained specialist in obstetric anaesthesia is an essential condition for the newborn.

CONCLUSION

It can be said that although gaps persist in our knowledge of this subject, many 'how and why' were answered. The problem is very complex, but, when we speak over the influence on the foetus of a drug administered to the mother, we must first consider what happens with the drug in the mothers organism, secondly how and how much it passes the placenta and only at last what happens with the drug in the foetal circulation and on which ground we can equivalent it to the adult dosage.

I think that we can best end these theoretical speculations with two practical thoughts:

– first, because so many influences and variables which are only partially known and under control, we have to give anaesthesia governed by the idea that unexpectedly big quantity of drugs can pass the placenta at one moment (1) and therefore it is more important how than what we give.

- second, we have not to forget that in obstetrics we are called to care for two patients but to anaesthetise only one.

Since the present communication was reported a small change of our anaesthetic technique for caesarean section was introduced. We prefer now to induce anaesthesia with propanidid (Epontol) which, beeing inactivated by placental cholin-estherase is much less depressant for the newborn as Pentothal.

REFERENCES

1. Marx G. F., Placental transfer and drugs used in anesthesia. *Anesthesiology* 22, 2, 294 (1961).
2. Walts L. F., Dillon J. B., The response of newborn to succinylcholine and d Tubocurarine. *Anesthesiology* 31, 1, 35 (1969).
3. Baker J. B. E., The effect of drugs on the foetus. *Pharmacol. Rev.* 12, 37 (1960).
4. Moya F., Thomdike V., Passage of drugs across the placenta. *Amer. J. Obstetr. Gynaec.* 84, 11/2, 1778 (1962).
5. Paton W. D. M., Principles of drug action. *Proc. Roy. Soc. Med.* 53, 815 (1960).
6. Price H. L., A dynamic concept of the distribution of thiopental in the human body. *Anesthesiology,* 21, 1, 40 (1960).
7. Selwyn-Crawford J., Rudofski S., The significance of varying the mode of administration of a drug. *Brit. J. Anaesth.* 38, 8, 628 (1966).
8. Selwyn-Crawford J., Rudofski S., The mode of administration of Promazine as a factor in determining the extent placental transmission. *Brit. J. Anaesth.* 37, 5, 310 (1965).
9. Selwyn-Crawford J., Rudofski S., The placental transmission of pethidine. *Brit. J. Anaesth.* 37, 12, 929 (1965).
10. Thomas J. et al., The placental transfer of Alcuronium. *Brit. J. Anaesth.* 4, 41, 297 (1969).
11. Kirby D. R. S., *Transplantation and pregnancy in human transplantation* (Rappaport, Dausset). Grune & Stratton, New York 1968.
12. Moya F., Thomdike V., The effects of drugs used in labor on the foetus and newborn. *Clin. Pharmac. Ther.* 4, 5, 628 (1963).
13. Bernstine R. L., Placental capicity and its relationship to foetal health. *Clin. Obstetr. Gynaec.* 3, 853 (1960).
14. Reynolds, Regulation of foetal circulation. *Clin. Obstetr. Gyn.* 3, 834 (1960).
15. Older P. O., Harris J. M., Placental transfer of tubocurarine. *Brit. J. Anaesth.* 40, 6, 459 (1968).
16. Adriani J., Placental transfer of local anesthetic drugs. *Appraisal Curr. Conc. Anesthesia.* 4, 178 (1968).
17. Apgar V., Holaday D. A. et al., Comparison of regional and general anesthesia in obstetrics. *J.A.M.A.* 165, 17, 2155 (1957).
18. Adriani J., Interaction of Magnesium ion with anesthetic drugs. *Appraisal Curr. Conc. Anesth.* 4, 124 (1968).
18. Gordon H. R. Fatal bradycardia after paracervical block. *New. Engl. J. Med.* 279, 10, 910 (1968).

19. Epstein B. S. et al., Comparative effects of Prilocaine and Lidocaine during peridural anesthesia for obstetrics. *An. & An. C.R.* 47, 3, 228 (1968).
20. Schnider J. M., Leong Way E., The kinetics of transfer of lidocaine across the human placenta. *Anesthesiology* 29, 5, 9, 44 (1968).
21. Churchill-Davidson H. C., Wise R. P., Neuromuscular transmission in the newborn infant. *Anesthesiology* 24, 271 (1963).
22. Hehre F. W., Continuous lumbar peridural anaesthesia in obstetrics. *An. & An. C.R.* 48, 2, 177 (1969).
23. Shnider J. M., Leong Way E., Plasma levels of lidocaine in mother and newborn following obstetrical conduction anesthesia. *Anesthesiology* 29, 5, 951 (1968).
24. Williams B., The present place of spinal subarachnoid analgesia in obstetrics. *Brit. J. Anaesth.* 41, 7, 628 (1969).
25. Lerner S. M. et al., Anesthetic considerations for complicated obstetrics. *An. & An. C.R.* 48, 5, 771 (1969).
26. Barklay D. L. et al., The influence of inferior vena cava compression on the level of spinal anesthesia. *Amer. J. Obstetr Gynaec.* 101, 7, 792 (1968).
27. Bromage P. R., Spread of analgesic solutions in the epidural space and their site of action. *Brit. J. Anaesth.* 34, 3, 161 (1962).
28. Marx G. F., Orkin L. R., Cerebrospinal fluid proteins and spinal anesthesia in obstetrics. *Anesthesiology* 26, 3, 340 (1965).
29. Bessem N. D., *De keizersnede*. Proefschrift, Leiden 1969.
30. Epstein B. S. et al., Passage of Lidocaine and Prilocaine across the placenta. *An. & An. C.R.,* 47, 3, 223 (1968).
31. Gunther R. E., Bauman J., Obstetrical caudal anesthesia. *Anaesthesia* 31, 1, 5 (1969).
32. John A. H., Placental transfer of Atropine. *Brit. J. Anaesth.* 37, 1, 57 (1965).
33. Levy C. J., Owen G., Thiopentone transmission through placenta. *Anaesthesia* 19, 4, 511 (1964).
34. Moya F., Smith B. E., Uptake distribution and placental transport of drugs and anesthetics. *Anesthesiology* 26, 4, 465 (1965).
35. Selwyn-Crawford J., Rudofski S., Placental transmission and neonatal metabolism of Promazine. *Brit. J. Anaesth.* 37, 5, 303 (1965).

THE INFLUENCE OF ANESTHESIA ON THE
ACID-BASE VALUES OF MOTHER AND CHILD

J. SPIERDIJK

The knowledge of the anaesthetist can support the team in the delivery-room. Not only in cases when the mother needs some kind of anaesthesia, but also with his knowledge of resuscitation. In several cases of birth-asphyxia we were asked to help and so we became interested in the possibilities of the prevention of conditions which make resuscitation necessary. An analysis of the acid-base balance can give us a good evaluation of the existence of asphyxia. So we asked ourselves is there an influence of the mother in the acid-base balance of the foetus, and secondly, what is the influence of anaesthesia in the acid-base values of that foetus.

Of importance are not only the anaesthetic drugs which as Dr. Popescu had mentioned, can have some depressing effects in the newborn, but also the technic used by the anaesthesiologist.

To describe changes in the acid-base balance of the body fluids we use the terms 'acidosis' and 'alkalosis'. Acidosis is used to describe patients with an increased hydrogen ionconcentration in the blood, in other words with a pH below 7.36. Is the pH above 7.44 we use the term alkalosis. The change in hydrogen ionconcentration may occur as a result of a primary respiratory disturbance or as a primary metabolic disturbance.

We express the respiratory component in terms of pCO_2 and the metabolic component as positive or negative Base-Excess, where Base-Excess is defined as the titratable base on titration with strong acid to normal pH at normal pCO_2 and normal temperature.

A primary acid-base abnormality is countered initially by bufferreactions in blood. Buffers, by their presence in solution, minimise changes in pH to the addition of both acids and bases.

A secondary physiological process occurring in response to a primary disturbance in one component of acid-base equilibrium is called compensation. Here the component not primarily affected will change in such a direction as to restore blood pH to normal.

We are in this story especially interested in metabilic acidosis and respiratory alkalosis of the mother and in metabolic acidosis and respiratory acidosis of the child.

Metabolic acidosis is defined as a gain of strong acid or a loss of bicarbonate of the extra cellular fluid. The buffer-response to a metabolic acidosis is a fall in plasma bicarbonate, Base Excess is lower and pCO_2 is normal. The compensation of a metabolic acidosis is a respiratory one. This compensation will restore the pH to normal, the pCO_2 will fall. This process starts at once, but it takes 12 to 24 hours before maximal compensation is reached (fig. 1).

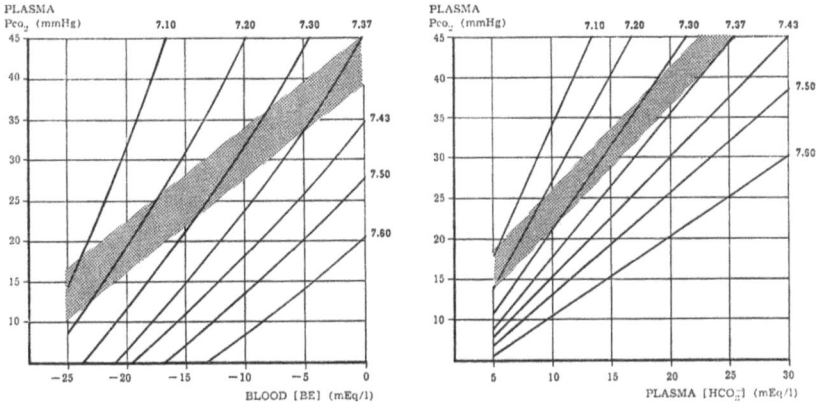

Fig. 1. Ninety-five percent confidence limits for maximally compensated sustained metabolic acidosis.

Respiratory acidosis is defined as an abnormal process in which there is a primary decrease in the rate of alveolar ventilation relative to the rate of CO_2-production.

The buffer-response is a fall in pH, an elevation of pCO_2 and a fall in B.E. (fig. 2 and 3). There is a fall in B.E. because bicarbonate diffuses from the blood into the interstitial fluid, according to Winters (1). The compensation is renal, H-ions are excreted and bicarbonate reabsorbed. Maximal compensation is reached after one to six days, the urine is acid (fig. 4). Respiratory alkalosis is defined as an abnormal physiological process in which there is a primary increase in the rate of alveolair ventilation relative to the rate of CO_2 production.

The buffer-response to a respiratory alkalosis is an increase in pH, a decrease in pCO_2 and an unaltered B.E. (fig. 5). The compensation, there

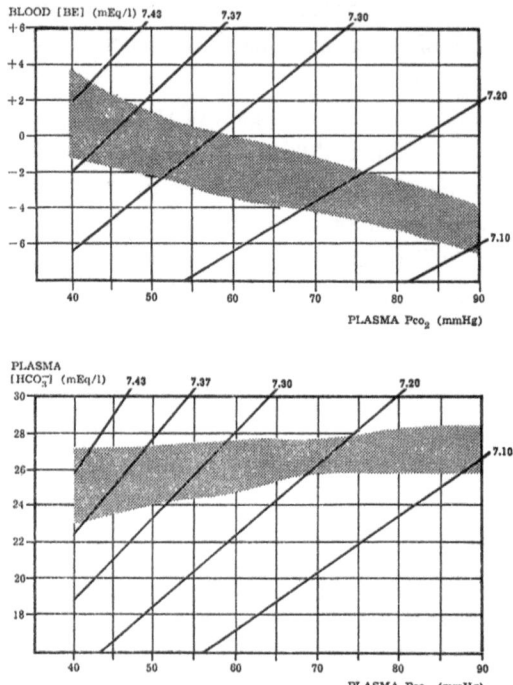

Fig. 2.   Ninety-five percent confidence limits for acute respiratory acidosis.

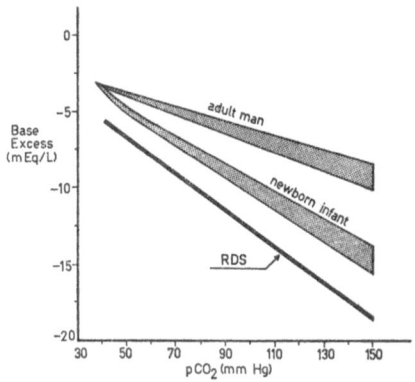

Fig. 3.   RDS data from Kildeberg, P., *Acta Ped.* 53, 505 (1964).
BE = –0.116 p CO_2–1.02, e = –0,73, n = 48.

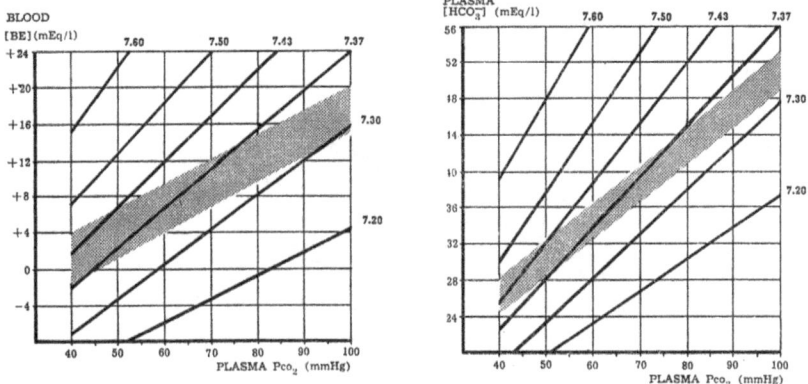

Fig. 4. Ninety-five percent confidence limits for maximally compensated sustained respiratory acidosis.

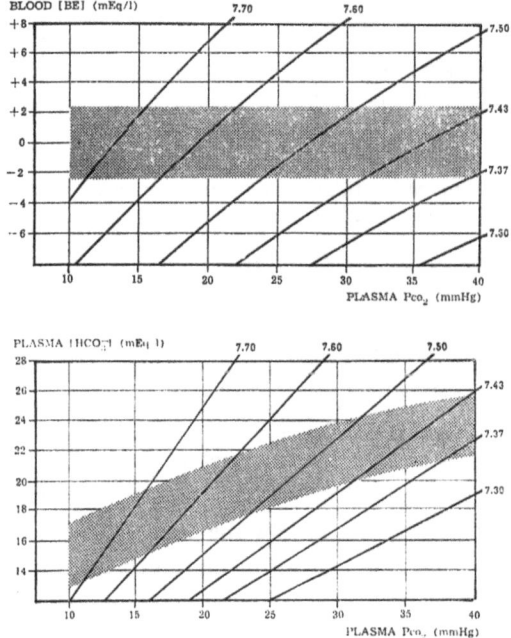

Fig. 5. Ninety-five percent confidence limits for acute respiratory alkalosis. (Constructed on the assumption that the *in vivo* response is the same as the *in vitro* response).

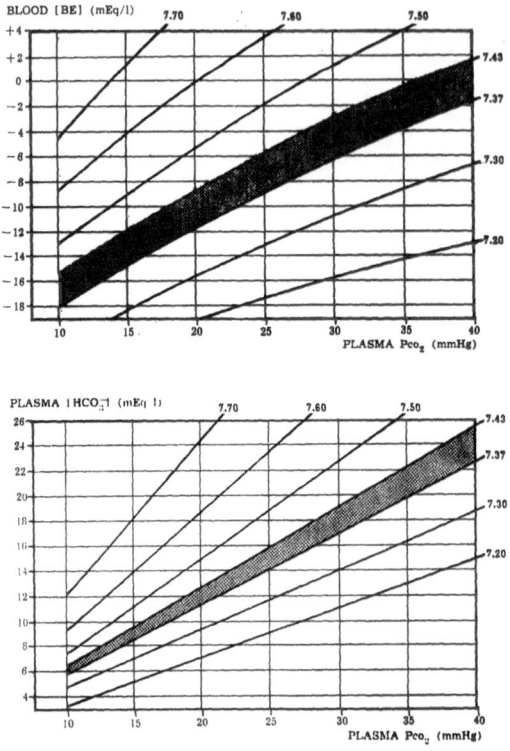

Fig. 6. Ninety-five percent confidence limits for maximally compensated sustained respiratory alkalosis. (Constructed on the assumption that blood pH is restored to normal).

is a loss of bicarbonate, the B.E. shall fall. The urine is alkaline, it takes 6 hours – 6 days (fig. 6 and 7).

Well, let us go back to the mother and the newborn. In 1961, Bruns, Cooper and Drose (2) reported the results of simultaneous measurements of oxygen tension, acid-base balance and hydrogen ionconcentrations in the pregnant mother and the foetus at the moment of birth. They conclude that a pregnant normal woman and the foetus in utero are apparently sufficiently well oxygenated and in an undisturbed acid-base equilibrium at the moment of delivery. In mothers with certain complications of pregnancy the foetus in utero has a measurable amount of respiratory and metabolic acidosis. Rooth in 1964 (3) observed a close correlation between the foetal and maternal metabolic acidosis. In order to evaluate foetal acidosis, it is enough to measure maternal acidosis. He says: the onset of

Fig. 7

	Metabolic acidosis		
Acute → buffer response	pH ↓	BE ↓	pCO₂ normal
Sustained → compensation 0–24 hrs.	pH ↑	BE ↓	pCO₂ ↓
	Respiratory acidosis		
Acute → bufferresponse	pH ↓	pCO₂ ↑	BE ↓
Sustained → compensation 1–6 days	pH ↑	pCO₂ ↑	BE ↑
	Respiratory Alkalosis		
Acute → buffer response	pH ↑	pCO₂ ↓	BE normal
Sustained → compensation 6 hrs–6 days	pH ↓	pCO₂ ↓	BE ↓

maternal metabolic acidosis can be gauged by the intensity and the frequency of pains. Maternal and foetal acidosis, therefore predominantly results from labour at the time when the maternal muscular efforts become so great that the oxygen demand by her working tissues can not be met. Beard and Morris (4) also observed that the progressive maternal metabolic acidosis if excessive, may depress the condition of the baby at birth, despite and adequate placental exchange. Saling (5), Beard and Morris (4), Kubli and Berg (6) and Eckenhausen (7) have evaluated the acid-base equilibrium by means of obtaining capillary blood from the presenting part of the foetus in utero. During labour the writers have observed a decrease in foetal pH and base-excess and a rise in pCO_2. Kubli and Berg (6) don't think that the maternal acidosis accounts for the pathological foetal acidosis, accompanying foetal distress.

The metabolic acidosis in the foetus is in the first place an indication of an anaerobic metabolism. It is evidence of oxygen supply to the foetus that was not optimal. Secondly it is possible that there is a disturbance in the exchange of hydrogen ions and lactate from the foetus to the mother. Thirdly, as we have mentioned, a metabolic acidosis of the mother could be transferred to the foetus. And at last, we have to deal with the hyperventilation of the mother. As we have seen before, the full compensation of an hyperventilation can give the same acid-base values as gives the full compensation of a metabolic acidosis.

Hyperventilation occurs in many women during labour, it is a part of the technique for painless childbirth, or occur spontaneously by pain, apprehension and anxiety.

It is of interest to know if we have to deal with a primary metabolic acidosis of the mother (caused by muscular work and starvation during labour) or we have to deal with a primary respiratory alkalosis (due to hyperventilation). Of 12 mothers we obtained the acid-base values before, during and after labour. During the first part of labour in all cases we saw a slight increase in pH and a decrease in pCO_2. The B.E. decreases or remains unaltered. During the second part of labour, the pH decreased, the pCO_2 increased and the B.E. decreased (fig. 8 and 9).

This is accordingly to the figures of Beard and Morris (4). So, the

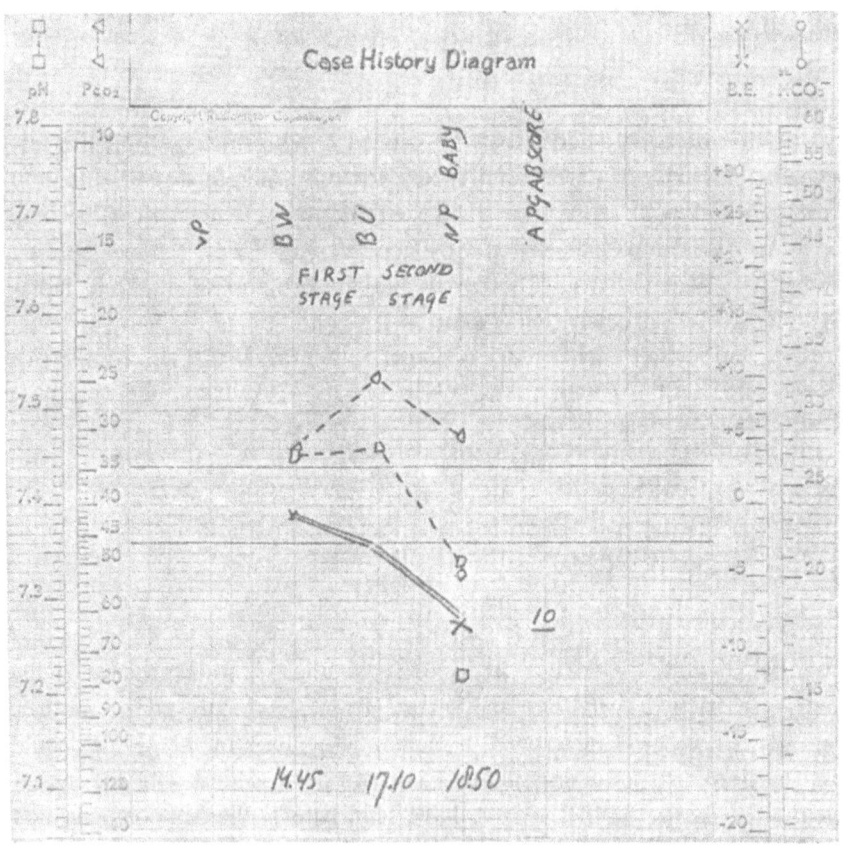

Fig. 8

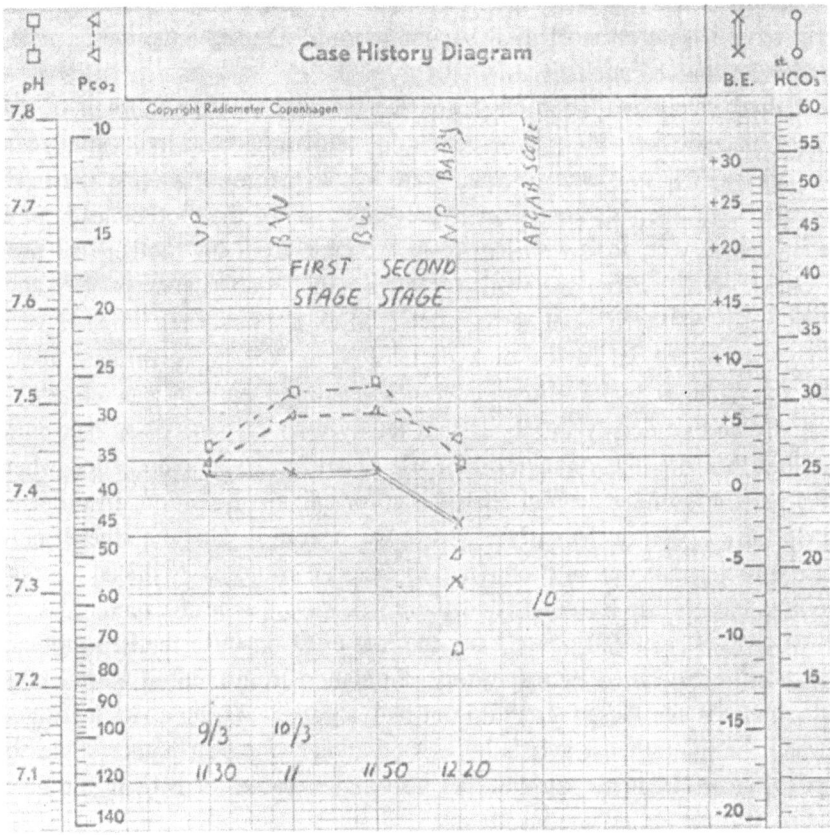

Fig. 9

possibilities exists that in the first stage of labour we have to deal with a primary hyperventilation, in long term cases leading to a loss of bicarbonate and in the second stage we have to deal with a metabolic acidosis caused by muscular work. Most of the times, labour is going on and there is no time that hyperventilating patients can develop a compensatory metabolic acidosis, losing bicarbonate.

We started to observe the urine pH in portions to confirm this hypothesis. As preliminary communication (we have had only 5 patients), I told of four patients the urine was acid. One had an alkaline urine, this was a woman, not in labour, waiting the night in the hospital for a caesarean section. The pCO_2 decreased from 35.0 till 30.5, the pH unchanged 7.47, B.E. from + 1.9 till − 0.6. She was hyperventilating during more than

12 hours. The baby was born with a pH of 7.10, pCO_2 88.1, B.E. −8.9 and oxygen saturation of 49.8, Apgar score 9! During anaesthesia pCO_2 and pH remained unchanged.

I think hyperventilation can influence the acid-base equilibrium of the foetus in two ways. First: hyperventilation and subsequent hypocapnia can impair the transplacental oxygen transport as Motoyama et al (8) have pointed out. Second: long term hyperventilation of the mother leads to a compensatory acidosis with loss of bicarbonate from the mother and also from the child. From the work of Moya and his colleagues (9) it seems that the critical level of maternal arterial pCO_2 is 17 mm Hg, this is a very low level of arterial carbon-dioxyde tension, unlikely to be brought about by spontaneous hyperventilation. But some upset patients can breath so rapidly and so deeply in labour that tetany with carpopedal spasme may follow. A more likely danger is the use of artificial hyperventilation when the patient is under general anaesthesia for caesarean section. In order to help the surgeon in the early stages of the operation, the anaesthetist may use muscle relaxants in preference to deep anaesthesia. Artificial ventilation is part of the technique and there is always a risk of overventilation.

As Moya et al. (9) pointed out the low pCO_2 in unaesthetised mothers is most likely caused by respiratory stimulation from painfull uterine contractions. When these factors do not play a part as during anaesthesia and when the anaesthetist avoids hyperventilation we expect higher values of pCO_2 and B.E. in the mother and also higher values of B.E. in the newborn, if there are no complications.

At 36 normal deliveries without analgesia we obtained one minute after birth, the Apgar score and by means of the micro Astrup technique the acid-base values of mother (fingerprick) and child (heelprick).

Of 24 caesarean sections we obtained the same values. I present the mean values of pH, pCO_2 and B.E. of 36 mothers and their babies in table 1. Of interest are the last two babies with the low Apgar score. The last one had a Base-Excess of minus twenty point zero. The value of the mother was minus six point zero. It was a 'breech delivery' and there must have been a disturbance in the oxygenation of the child.

The child with an Apgar score of four had a Base-Excess of minus eighteen point six. This value in the mother was minus ten point six. This was also a breech delivery, with the possibility of a disturbance in the oxygenation of the child. However an other mechanism can play a part. Metabolic acidosis of the mother can give here a metabolic acidosis of the child. And thirdly a primary sustained respiratory alkalosis of the mother can have had its influence on the child. The origin of the low B.E. in this child lies I think in a hyperventilation of the mother.

Here I present the Astrup values and the Apgar score of 24 caesarean sections (table 2). The patients were breathing spontaneously and were not intubated. Until the baby was born a cyclo-oxygen mixture, followed by nitrogen-oxydyle-oxygen mixture was given by a Waters-system without absorbtion of CO_2. When we compare the spontaneous born group with a high Apgar score and the caesarean section group, we see the following values (table 3). It seems to be that there is no influence of anaesthesia in the acid-base balance of the vigorous newborn. You can see that there

Table 1. 36 Patients apgar score and mean acid-base values.

Patients	Apgar score	Mother			Child		
		pH	pCO_2	BE	pH	pCO_2	BE
17	10	7.41	30.9	− 3.6	7.21	57.9	− 5.9
16	9	7.40	28.6	− 5.4	7.18	61.6	− 8.7
1	6	7.41	33.8	− 2.1	7.24	59.0	− 5.8
1	4	7.35	22.2	−10.6	7.04	60.8	−18.6
1	2	7.38	30.1	− 6.0	6.91	70.0	−20.0

Table 2. 24 Caesarean sections.

Patients	Apgar Score	Mother			Child		
		pH	pCO_2	B.E.	pH	pCO_2	B.E.
9	10	7.36	39.4	−2.9	7.21	56.0	− 6.8
9	9	7.36	37.8	−3.8	7.20	57.9	− 7.3
2	6	7.36	37.3	−3.4	7.12	67.4	− 8.8
2	4	7.34	42.1	−3.6	7.11	65.8	−10.1
2	2	7.25	53.4	−5.2	7.02	70.0	−13.8

Table 3.

	Patients	Apgar Score	Mother			Child		
			pH	pCO_2	B.E.	pH	pCO_2	B.E.
Normal	33	9–10	7.41	29.7	−4.5	7.19	59.7	−7.3
Caesarean Sections	18	9–10	7.36	38.6	−3.3	7.20	57.0	−7.0

Table 4. Caesarean sections Apgar Score < 9.

Apgar score	pat. no.	Mother			Child			Indication Caesarean section	Cause low score	Score after 10 min.
		pH	pCO$_2$	B.E.	pH	pCO$_2$	B.E.			
6	72	7.37	40.2	−1.8	7.12	62.8	− 7.7	contracted pelvis	anaesthesia	10
6	73	7.36	34.5	−5.0	7.12	72.0	−10.0	contracted pelvis	anaesthesia	10
4	48	7.40	34.2	−3.0	7.13	66.0	−10.1	vaginal prolapse	anaesthesia	10
4	74	7.27	50.0	−4.2	7.08	65.7	−10.2	contracted pelvis	unknown	10
2	19	7.29	53.0	−3.9	7.18	62.0	− 9.6	preeclampsia	preeclampsia	6
2	71	7.21	59.9	−6.3	6.87	78.0	−18.1	preeclampsia	preeclampsia	4

is no influence of a moderate hyperventilation of the mother on the spontaneous born group. The following figure gives information about six caesarean sections with low Apgar scores (table 4). Three times the anaesthesia was not smooth. As you see the low pH of these children was caused by a higher pCO$_2$ and lower B.E. Further you see that in cases of placenta-insuffiency, the acidosis is more pronounced and the recovery of the children more difficult.

CONCLUSION

We observed the acid-base values of 77 women and their babies. In 12 cases we tried to follow the acid-base changes during labour, in 5 cases also with values of urine pH. Of sixty deliveries (36 spontaneously and 24 caesarean sections) we obtained one minute after birth the acid-base values of mother and child. Only in one case there was the possibility that hyperventilation of the mother was leading to foetal acidosis. When the anaesthesia was smooth, we saw no influence on Apgar scores and Astrup values. It is possible that during long lasting labour, hyperventilation of the mother leads to a serious metabolic acidosis of the child. Perhaps that in cases of caesarean section, hyperventilation by an anaesthetist aggravates this acidosis. Of more importance seems the fact that hyperventilation leads to a disturbance in the oxygen supply of the child by means of a reduction of the blood flow in the uterine arteria or placenta. So it is necessary that the anaesthetist avoids hyperventilation in his technique, especially in cases of long lasting labour and in cases of placenta insuffiency.

Thanks are extended to Miss H. van Meeverden and Dr. A. G. Zwart Voorspuy of the department of biochemistry and L. J. Wiersma of the department of gynaecology for their help and advice.

Figs. 1, 2, 4, 5 and 6 from: Winters, R. W., *Acid base physiology in medicine.* The London Company, Cleveland O, 1969.

REFERENCES

1. Winters R. W., *Acid-base fysiology in medecine.* London Company of Cleveland (1966).
2. Bruns P. D., Cooper W. E. and Drose V. E., Maternal-fetal oxygen and acid-base studies and their relationships to hyaline membrane disease in the newborn infant. *Amer. J. Obst. and Gyn.* 1079–82 (1961).
3. Rooth G., Early detection and prevention of foetal acidosis. *Lancet* 290 (1964).
4. Beard R. W. and Morris E. D., Foetal and maternal acid-base balance during normal labour. *J. Obst. and Gyn. Brit. Cwlth.* 496 (1965).
5. Saling E., *Das Kind im Bereich der Geburtshilfe.* Georg Thieme Verlag, Stuttgart.
6. Kubli F. and Berg D., The early diagnosis of foetal distress. *J. Obst. and Gyn. Brit. Cwlth.* 507 (1965).
7. Eckenhausen F. W., A study of the perinatal acid-base equilibrium. Thesis, Leiden (1969).
8. Motoyama E. K., Rivard G., Acheson F. and Cook C. D., Adverse effect of maternal hyperventilation on the foetus. *Lancet,* 286 (1966).
9. Moya F., Morishima H. O., Shnider S. M. and James L. S., Influence of maternal hyperventilation on the newborn infant. *Amer. J. Obst. and Gyn.* 1–76 (1965).

LITERATURE

Annotations, Hyperventilation and foetal acidosis. *Lancet* 1401 (1966).
Apgar V., Proposal for a new method of evaluation of newborn infants. *Anest. and Analg.* 32–260 (1953).
Apgar V., Infant resuscitation. *Post grad. Med.* 447 (1956).
Astrup P., Jørgensen K., Siggaard-Andersen O. and Engel K., The acid-base metabolism. A new approach. *Lancet* 1733 (1960).
Bruyne de J. J., De hypoxemische pasgeborene. *Ned. T. Geneesk.* 1985 (1965).
Coleman A. J., Absence of harmful effect of maternal hypocapnia in babies delivered at caesarean-section. *Lancet* 813 (1967).
Derom R. M., Maternal acid-base balance during labour. *Clin. obst. and Gyn.* vol. 110 (1968).
Eichenholz A., Mulhausen R. O., Anderson W. E. and MacDonald F. M. (1962). Primary hypocapnia: a cause of metabolic acidosis. *J. appl. Physiol.* 283–288 (1962).

Fischer W. M., Untersuchungen zum Säure/Bose-Gleichgewicht im fetalen Blut vor der Geburt. *Arch. Gyn.* 200 (1964).

Morishima M., Daniel S., Adamsons K. and James L. T., Effects of positive pressure ventilation of the mother upon the acid-base state of the fetus. *Amer. J. Obst. and Gyn.* 93–269 (1965).

Papadopoulos C. N. and Keats A. S., The metabolic acidosis of hyper-ventilation produced by controlled respiration. *Anaesthesiology* 20–156 (1959).

Rooth G. and Nilsson I., Studies on foetal and maternal metabolic acidosis. *Clin. Aci.* 26, 121–132 (1964).

Sikkel A., Intra-uterine hypoxemie. *Ned. Tijdschr. Geneesk.,* 1983 (1965).

Spierdijk J., Astrupwaarden bij moeder en pasgeborene. *Ned. Tijdschr. Geneesk.,* 1390 (1967).

Usher R., Mclean F. and Maughan G. B., Respiratory distress syndrome in infants delivered by Caesarean section. *Amer. J. Obst. Gyn.* 806 (1964).

Winters R. W., Studies of acid-base disturbances. *Pediatrics* vol. 39–5 (1967).

Wulf H., The oxygen and carbon dioxide tension gradients in the human placenta at term. *Am. J. Obst. Gyn.* 1–38 (1964).

TREATMENT OF ASPHYXIA OF THE NEWBORN

J. H. RUYS

Asphyxia in the newborn indicates a condition, which is characterized by hypoxaemia, acidosis and, usually, hypercapnia. The gravity of the asphyxia can only partially be judged by the degree of the disturbance of the acid-base equilibrium (1). During a normal delivery there appears to be a partial asphyxia in the fetus. This is shown in figure 1, derived from the study of Eckenhausen (2). It is generally accepted, that this condition of partial asphyxia after delivery, is the most important stimulus for the initiation of spontaneous breathing. But otherwise it is known, that fetal lambs, delivered by caesarean section and with intact umbilical circulation, can be stimulated to breath, merely by strong cooling and without change in acid-base equilibrium (3). In the human newborn, the clamping of the umbilical cord does not play an important part in the onset of breathing. Most newborns already breath before the clamping of the cord. But why

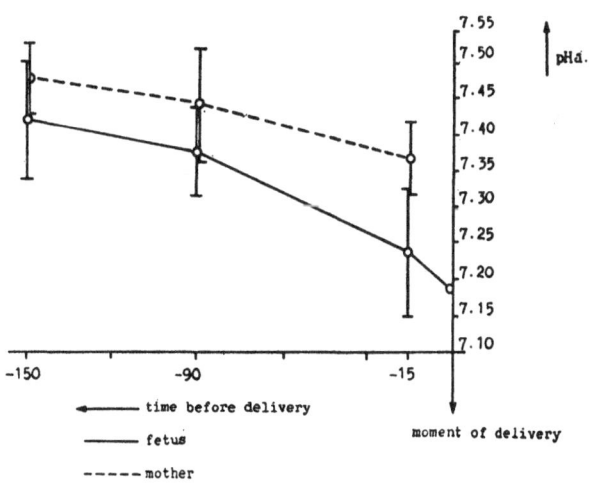

Fig. 1. Course of the actual pH of mother and child during labour until the moment of delivery (after Eckenhausen, 1969).

103

does respiration not start during delivery, whereas a partial asphyxia is already present in this period? There are indications from animal experiments that the carotid chemoreceptors are more or less inactive before birth (4) and are stimulated after birth by increased cervical sympathetic activity. The next question to be answered now, is, by what means the sympathetic nerves are stimulated after birth. As far as I know no special investigations have been done on this subject. There are several arguments in favour of a stimulation by cold stress. In conclusion the cold stimulus might play a primary part in the onset of breathing in the newborn before the clamping of the umbilical cord.

In spite of the onset of respiration, the deviations of acid-base equilibrium are increasing during the first 5–10 minutes after birth and are only gradually decreasing during the following 1–2 hours of life. Figure 2, derived from Eckenhausen (2), illustrates this sequence of events. This condition of protracted acidosis may have important consequences, especially in premature infants, for the respiratory function and for the resistance to early stress conditions.

After this introduction, I would like to discuss several kinds and causes of asphyxia and elucidate our methods of treatment in the Neonatal Unit of the Obstetric Department. The subjects are:

1.   Complete asphyxia with apnoea, immediately after delivery.
2.   Partial asphyxia without apnoea, and characterized by respiratory and/or metabolic acidosis.

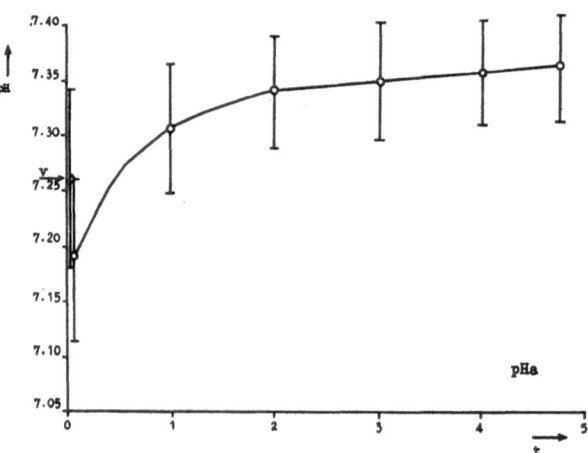

Fig. 2. Graph of the acid-base parameters determined hourly in heel blood means and standard deviations (after Eckenhausen, 1969).

3. Asphyxia (attacks of apnoea) sooner or later after delivery, by other causes:
   a. immaturity,
   b. hypoglycaemia,
   c. perforation of a subependymal haemorrhage,
   d. iatrogenically induced apnoeic attacks.

ad 1. COMPLETE ASPHYXIA WITH APNOEA, AFTER DELIVERY

Almost 10% of all newborns, admitted to the Neonatal Unit, had an Apgar Score of 3 or less and did not start breathing spontaneously, immediately after birth. The several causes for this state of depression, like intra-uterine hypoxaemia and mechanical birth injury are well known. After the delivery of such a newborn, we usually do not know if the child is in a state of primary or secondary apnoea.

The sequence of events during asphyxia is shown in figure 3, derived from experimental work of Dawes (3). Asphyxia starts with a period of primary apnoea, accompanied by a fall in heart rate. During this period, hypoxaemia and hypercapnia bring about a powerful stimulation of the chemoreceptors; moreover, there is an excess of external stimuli.

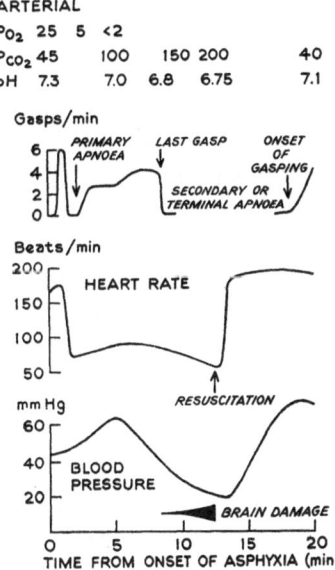

Fig. 3. Schematic diagram of changes in rhesus monkeys during asphyxia and on resuscitation by positive pressure ventilation. Brain damage was assessed by histological examination some weeks or months later (after Dawes, 1968).

All methods of resuscitation, with the intention to stimulate the respiratory centre (for instance with dimethylamide) or to stimulate cutaneous
receptors (for instance warm and cold tubbing) are superfluous and useless,
because, after the period of primary apnoea, always a period of gasping
ensues, as is shown in figure 3. If the airways are clear, gasping usually
will give rise to the onset of rhythmic breathing. If the child, however, was
already in the next period of secondary apnoea, immediately after delivery,
accompanied by a drop in blood pressure, and brain damage, then the
above mentioned methods are only harmful and a waste of time.

The only effective methods of resuscitation can be shortly outlined as
follows:

1. Clearing of the airways; if possible endotracheal suction should be
applied, but only by experienced people.

2. Oxygen administration by means of mouth-to-mouth ventilation; pay
attention to the right position of the head in retroflection; otherwise the air
entry is impeded.

If no rapid improvement is achieved, intubation should be performed,
followed by some kind of artificial ventilation. In the Neonatal Unit the
Amsterdam Infant Ventilator is always ready for use. To-day every resident in obstetrics and pediatrics should meet the requirement to obtain
experience in intubation.

3. Correction of acidosis, immediately after the first resuscitative measures, preferably with sodium bicarbonate 8,4%, combined with an equal
amount of glucose 10%. Without a preceding determination of the degree
of acidosis we feel justified in administering immediately 3 mEq sodium
bicarbonate per kg body-weight.

After a following determination of the acid-base state a further correction may be found necessary. Rapid correction is very important, because
the acidosis brings about a pulmonary vasoconstriction which prevents an
effective oxygen uptake. We must be aware that after administration of
sodium bicarbonate the acid-base values do not reflect anymore the clinical
condition of the newborn.

4. Protection against cooling during resuscitation is very important.
Under normal delivery room conditions deep body temperature of the
newborn falls 2 or 3 degrees Centigrade (fig. 4). Metabolic rate is increased 2–3 times upon exposure to cold, corresponding with an equal
increase in oxygen consumption.

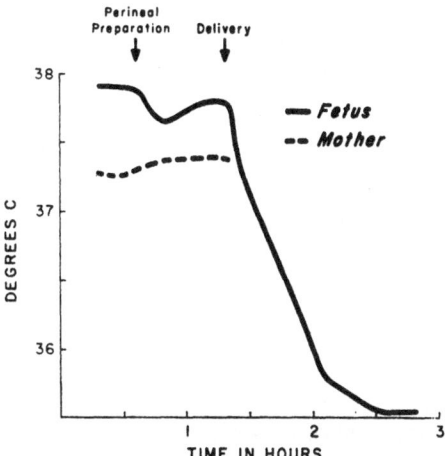

Fig. 4. Colonic temperatures of mother and fetus during labor and that of the newborn after delivery. (From Adamsons and Towell: *Anesthesiology*, 26:531, 1965. By courtesy of the J. B. Lippincott Company).

5. Cardiac massage may be necessary if the blood pressure is unduly low at the beginning of resuscitation. It should be instituted only, if a heart beat cannot be detected, or if the heart rate does not rise promptly after the lungs have been well expanded.

ad 2. PARTIAL ASPHYXIA WITHOUT APNOEA

If an infant has been born with preceding signs of intra-uterine hypoxaemia and/or with an Apgar Score of 7 or less and/or with a low birth weight, a determination of pH, pCO_2 and derived values should be performed. As we have already discussed, a certain degree of acidosis is normally seen after each delivery. What are the ultimate values, below which treatment is indicated? We consider a pH-value below 7.20 and a base excess below −10 as pathological values.

Therefore the indication for chemical correction depends upon the clinical condition of the infant (his Apgar Score), the degree of acidosis and his birth weight. In very small premature babies, especially with a birth weight below 1500 g, we will try to correct a smaller degree of acidosis too. One-third of all newborns, admitted to the Neonatal Unit in 1968, had an AS of 7 or less.

The interest of rapid chemical correction of acidosis is, among other things, to combat the pulmonary vasoconstriction. Pulmonary hypoperfusion may play an important part in the development of hyaline membrane disease in premature infants. Therefore early correction of acidosis seems to be of interest in the prevention of this disease.

Table 1 shows the autopsy findings in the 17 cases of death in the Neonatal Unit in 1968. There were only 4 cases of uncomplicated hyaline membrane disease and 3 cases of HMD combined with other causes of death, intracranial haemorrhage and fetal hydrops. Three of these 7 cases of HMD concerned immature infants. May be there is a correlation between this low incidence of hyaline membrane disease and the way of treatment. A second point of interest regarding early correction of acidosis, is to provide the already depressed infant a higher resistance against other influences (like hypoglycaemia and hypothermia), which oncemore may give rise to the development of acidosis.

The treatment of partially asphyxiated newborns in the Neonatal Unit consists of the following measures:

1. Correction of acidosis with NaHCO₃ 8,4%, with equal amounts of glucose 10%: injection or infusion in the umbilical vein.

In borderline cases the intragastric route may be used. Figure 5

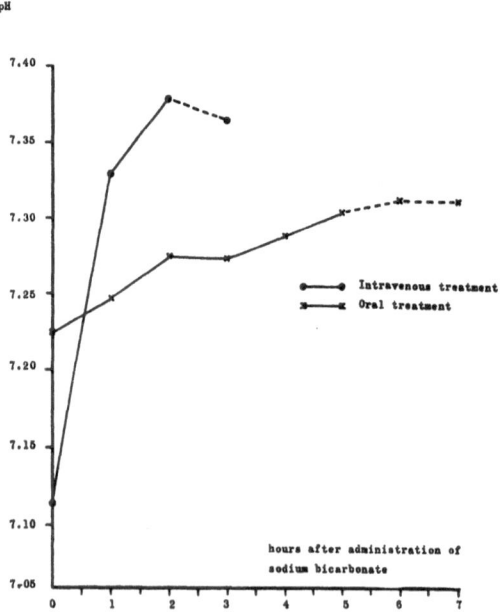

Fig. 5. Changes in mean pH-values in newborns with metabolic acidosis after intravenous or oral treatment with sodium bicarbonate.

Table 1. Neonatal mortality, neonatal unit, 1968.

Groups	Number of patients	Number of deaths	Autopsy findings							No autopsy
			HMD	ICH + HMD	ICH + HMD + HF	ICH	Hydrops fetalis	Atelectase	MCA	
Immaturity	8	6	1	2		1				2
Prematurity										
< 1000 g	1									
1000–1500 g	9	1							1	
1500–2000 g	30	4	1			1	1	1		
2000–2500 g	35 } 111	1	1							
2500–3000 g	27	1			1					
3000–3500 g	6									
> 3500 g	3									
Small for dates prematures	6	1							1	
Low birth weight at term	39									
Full term (excl. social indications)	72	3	1			2				
Postmaturity	7									
Total	243	17	4	2	1	4	1	1	2	2

Neonatal mortality (excl. immaturity) 46,8‰.

demonstrates, that correction of pH follows much more rapidly after intra-venous administration. If the total amount of $NaHCO_3$ did not exceed 10 mEq/kg body-weight/3 hours, I never noticed an important rise in serum sodium level. The infusion of a hypertonic solution gives rise to a rapid osmotic dilution of the blood and there may be brought about a striking hypoproteinaemia. The use of THAM solution has been aban-doned in our department.

2. Next to the correction of acidosis, small premature infants and low birth weight infants at term, are provided with an infusion of glucose 10%.

3. Oxygen administration is regularly checked by determination of the oxygen content in the incubator air by means of an oxygen analyzer. Failures in oxygen supply to the incubator can be detected rapidly in this way.

4. Careful temperature regulation of the incubator in – what we sup-pose to be – the so-called neutral temperature zone of the newborn. Precise information about the so-called set-point of the critical tempera-ture, the lower limit of the neutral temperature zone, at various weight and gestational age is scarce (5, 6, 7). Moreover with the commercial in-cubator, the adjustment of the air temperature to secure the supposed neutral zone, will often be insufficient to get the lowest possible metabolic rate, because there may be large differences in ambient temperature by radiant heat loss.

5. Regular control of acid-base equilibrium, oxygen saturation or pO_2 and the radiologic aspect of the lungs and the heart configuration. A metabolic acidosis, resistant to buffering treatment, is a sign of persisting hypoxaemia and an indication for artificial ventilation.

ad 3. ASPHYXIA (APNOEIC ATTACKS) BY OTHER CAUSES

a. *Immaturity* may be the cause. If the apnoeic attacks in immature in-fants are not brought about by complications, like intracranial haemor-rhage or hyaline membrane disease, the chance of surviving is dependent, to a large extent, upon the supervision and monitoring. The best monitor is a good nurse.

Most of the commercial respiration monitors are not adapted to im-mature and premature infants. Thermistors in the nostrils are impracticable on account of fastening problems and because a high incubator tempera-ture gives too slight a difference between in- and exspired air temperature. Expansion transducers with a microswitch turned out to be of no use in these small infants. Till now the registration of impedance through the thoracic cage has given the most satisfactory results; the fastening of the electrodes can be better accomplished with ordinary adhesive plaster than with the original double adhesive rings.

Registration of the abdominal wall movements during respiration with a foto-electrical cell seems to be a rewarding development in monitoring. The transmission of the impulse to the foto-electrical cell by means of a sewing thread is not yet full-proof, but small improvements may be enough to make it a useful instrument.

Rapid and effective treatment of an apnoeic attack by the nurse on duty is very important. If cutaneous stimulation is not effective, she has to be trained to use the Pulmotor immediately; this is a simple artificial ventilator, working according to the Poliomat principle.

In the meantime, the resident in charge can be called up, and if necessary the decision can be made for intubation and artificial ventilation with the Amsterdam Infant Ventilator.

b. An other cause of apnoeic attacks beside immaturity is hypoglycaemia. Dr. de Leeuw will discuss this subject more fully.

c. The third cause may be the perforation of a subependymal haemorrhage. This is of frequent occurrence on the first day of life (8), but according to my own experience a later and rather abrupt appearance is not seldom seen. Diagnosis can often be confirmed by performing a lumbar puncture; if there exists an obvious haemorrhage, further intervention is regarded as useless and even unjustifiable, in view of the very small chance of keeping this infant alive, and if so, resulting in a spastic, idiot child.

d. The last subject is the iatrogenically induced apnoeic attack. Some possibilities will be mentioned.

– The administration of THAM solution may induce an apnoeic attack: the accompanying fall of pCO_2 of short duration, implies a decrease of respiratory stimulation and may give rise to hypoventilation or even an apnoeic attack. That means, that it is incorrect to administer THAM solution without having the experience and possibilities for artificial ventilation of the infant.

– A second example. Phenobarbitone is used to treat convulsions in newborn infants, after exclusion of hypoglycaemia and hypocalcaemia as possible causes. If this treatment is unsuccessful, diazepam is often the drug of choice. One should be aware that phenobarbitone has a very long elimination time in the newborn and the combination with diazepam therapy introduces the danger of potentiating the central depressive activity, which may cause an apnoeic attack.

– A too high incubator temperature probably also may result in respiratory arrest. Figure 6 shows an observation of apnoeic attacks during a period of a too high incubator temperature.

In the introduction I already stressed the importance of the cold stimulus for the onset of breathing. Brück (5) demonstrated that, especially during the first day of life, the set-point for the critical temperature might be considerably lower in small premature babies than the generally used temperature range. Perlstein et al. (9) noticed, that apnoeic attacks occurred more frequently during the heating period of the incubator.

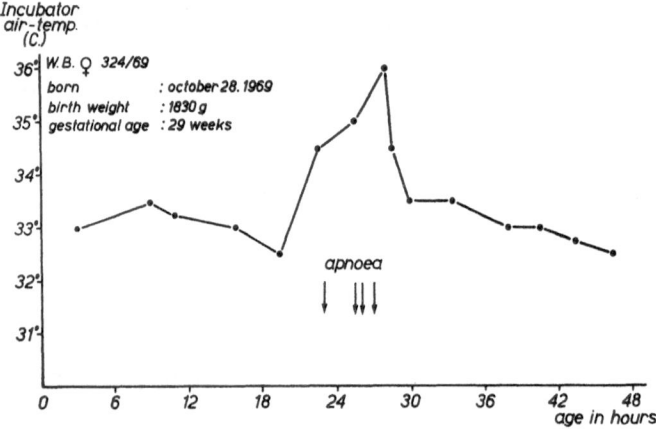

Fig. 6. Apnoeic attacks during an accidental increase in incubator air-temperature.

– Finally apnoeic attacks may occur during exchange transfusions. Presumably because the donor blood was too cold and the umbilical catheter had been pushed up too far in the direction of the heart, I noticed cardiac arhythmia in small premature babies during exchange transfusions. This might give rise to pulmonary and cerebral hypoperfusion with respiratory disturbances and even apnoeic attacks.

We are using now a specially built exchange transfusion table, with an electrically warmed, double walled trough and a radiant heat source above. Donor blood is prewarmed in a thermostatically controlled warm water basin. Rectal temperature and cardiac rate are continuously monitored. Artificial ventilation is immediately available.

All these measures in the treatment of asphyxia of the newborn do not alter the fact, that newborn infants, and especially premature infants, born with a low Apgar Score, have a high neonatal mortality rate. This may be shown in table 2, demonstrating the correlation between Apgar Score and neonatal mortality in the Neonatal Unit of this hospital in 1968. Ten percent of the newborns had an AS of 3 or less and a neonatal mortality of 35%; the newborns with an AS of 8–10 had a neonatal mortality of only 2,5%.

Table 2. Apgar Score and Neonatal Mortality. Neonatal Unit 1968.

Groups	number	0–3	Neon. †	4–7	Neon. †	8–10	Neon. †
				Apgar Score			
Immaturity	8	2	2	4	3	2	1
Prematurity							
<1000 g	1			1			
1000–1500 g	9	3	1	2		4	
1500–2000 g	30	3	2	10	1	17	1
2000–2500 g	35	1	1	5		29	
2500–3000 g	27	1	1	7		19	
3000–3500 g	6					6	
>3500 g	3			2		1	
	111	8	5	27	1	76	1
			62.5%		4%		1.3%
Small for dates prematures	6	2	1	1		3	
Low birth weight at term	39	2		5		32	
Full term (excl. social indications)	72	8		21	1	43	2
Postmaturity	7	1		2		4	
Total	243	23	8	60	5	160	4
			35%		8%		2.5%
Total, without immaturity	235	21	6	56	2	158	3
			29.6%		3.6%		1.9%
Neonatal mortality			4.7%				

The neonatal mortality on an average was 4,7% in the Neonatal Unit. The neonatal mortality in the whole Obstetric department was 6,4‰, which is lower than in the Netherlands as a whole. It is encouraging to reach such low values of neonatal mortality in a hospital, which attracts so much pathology.

REFERENCES

1. Frenzel J., Rogner G. und Maak B. Veränderungen des Lactat/Pyruvat-Quotienten bei hypoxischen Neugeborenen unter der Puffertherapie. *Monatsschr. Kinderheilk.* 116, 547 (1968).
2. Eckenhausen F. W. *A study of the perinatal acid-base equilibrium.* Thesis, Leiden 1969.
3. Dawes G. S. *Foetal and neonatal physiology.* Year Book Med. Publ. Chicago 1968.
4. Purves M. J. and Biscoe T. J. Development of chemoreceptor activity. *Brit. Med. Bull.* 22, 56 (1966).
5. Brück K. General aspects of temperature regulation of small subjects. In: *The adaptation of the newborn infant to extra-uterine life.* ed. J. H. P. Jonxis e.a. Stenfert Kroese, Leiden 1964.
6. Scopes J. W. Metabolic rate and temperature control in the human baby. *Brit. Med. Bull.* 22, 88 (1966).
7. Vlugt J. J. van der, *Studies on metabolic rate in low birth-weight infants.* Thesis, Groningen (1967).
8. Daamen C. B. F. *Perinatal mortality in Rotterdam.* Thesis, Leiden 1966.
9. Perlstein P. H., Edwards M. K. and Sutherland J. M. Apnea in premature infants as related to changes in environmental air temperatures (abstract). *Ped. Research* 3, 381 (1969).

THE INCIDENCE AND TREATMENT OF
HYPOGLYCEMIA IN THE NEWBORN

R. DE LEEUW

The occurrence of low glucose blood values in newborns has been known for some decades. In some cases one can find extremely low values (less than 20 mg%), we then speak of *neonatal hypoglycemia*. Sometimes this is attended by clinical symptoms as hypotonia, pallor, cyanosis, tremors or convulsions, in many cases however these symptoms are not found. Hypoglycemia with clinical symptoms in the newborn is called *symptomatic* neonatal hypoglycemia.

In general, hypoglycemia is a dangerous condition because of the danger of cerebral damage. The brain is probably entirely dependent on glucose for its metabolism. Cerebral symptoms may appear when the glucose concentration in the blood falls beneath a critical level. When this condition exists for a long time lasting cerebral damage may follow.

Newborn infants tolerate low glucose blood values better than older children and adults; cerebral symptoms usually appear later. The reason for this is not clear at the moment. Probably the brain of the newborn uses altered metabolic pathways or may use other sources of energy. However, serious symptomatic neonatal hypoglycemia leads to lasting cerebral damage in the majority of cases. In less serious and asymptomatic cases the outcome is not so clear. Nevertheless the development of the syndrome of minimal braindamage is by no means to be excluded. Certainly the most important factor in this is the duration of the hypoglycemia.

This is the reason why it is so difficult to assess the significance of neonatal hypoglycemia and to decide whether to treat it, or not.

The *pathogenesis* of neonatal hypoglycemia is very complicated (table 1). The parts played by the various factors involved have not been adequately explained. There is a balance of supply and removal of glucose in the body. Interference with this balance may result in hypoglycemia.

All newborn infants have a decreased hepatic output of glucose in the first hours after birth. This explains the initial temporary decrease of the

115

Table 1. Glucose homoiostasis in the newborn infant.

Supply of glucose	Removal of glucose
Hepatic output $\longrightarrow$ Glucose $\longrightarrow$ Peripheral use	
Glycogen-store	Glucose dependent tissues (brains)
Glycogen-breakdown	Other tissues
Gluconeogenesis	Metabolic rate
Glucose-release	Tissue oxygenation
Hormonal control	Availability of other Energy stores (lipolysis)
Feeding	Hormonal control (insulin)
Imbalance leads to hypoglycemia	

glucose content in the blood. A true hypoglycemic condition may originate if hepatic output is decreased more than normal, if peripheral use of glucose is sharply increased, or if there is no exogenous supply of glucose.

In certain pathological states the risk of neonatal hypoglycemia is increased, for instance in small-for-dates babies, babies of diabetic mothers, in cases of neonatal asphyxia, hypothermia etc.

The *incidence* of neonatal hypoglycemia is not exactly known for it depends on how careful it is looked for. Certainly it is not a rare condition. The composition of the studygroup (all newborns or only pathological cases) as well as the frequency of the glucose-determinations that have been done, are very important in estimating the incidence. In addition, the definition of hypoglycemia and the method of sampling and analyzing the blood for glucose are of considerable significance.

Comparing the statements about incidence of neonatal hypoglycemia made by different investigators is therefore a difficult problem. Recent studies give percentages of 5–15% of hypoglycemia in the admissions to a special care unit for newborns.

To get information about the incidence of neonatal hypoglycemia we studied in the Obstetric and Neonatal Department of the University of Amsterdam all newborns that we considered at risk (table 2). We did glucose determinations frequently from the moment of birth during the first 3–4 days. To facilitate making a survey we used the classification of newborn infants based on birth-weight and gestational age of Yerushalmy (1967).

In the one-year period september 1968 till september 1969 there were 1781 intra-mural newborns; in addition there were 61 newborns admitted in the first 48 hours of life from other hospitals or from home for various pathological conditions. Of a total of 1842 newborns in 531 cases (or about 30%) glucose-determinations were done. This group was considered 'at risk' for neonatal hypoglycemia.

We considered a condition hypoglycemic when a glucose concentration in the blood of 20 mg% or less was found. Others consider a newborn baby as hypoglycemic only, when there are two or more consecutive glucose values below 20 mg%. We think that as long as the significance of neonatal hypoglycemia is still so unclear one has to consider all infants with very low levels as hypoglycemic, even when one has only one value below 20 mg%. At least when the sampling and the method of analyzing of the blood for glucose are reliable. Because at this moment we cannot monitor the glucose blood content continuously we never know exactly how long the hypoglycemia has existed. How long a hypoglycemia may exist without producing brain-damage is fully unknown. Certainly not all these cases of hypoglycemia are serious and significant ones.

The percentage of hypoglycemic newborns in the 'at risk' group is very

Table 2. Incidence of neonatal hypoglycemia (Sept. 1, 1968–Aug. 31, 1969) Obstetric and neonatal department, University of Amsterdam.

I. Intramural	Total number	Glucose control = 'at risk'	Hypo- glycemia	Percen- tage of total	Percen- tage of 'at risk'
A. Very low birth weight <1500 g	34	16	6	18 %	38%
B. Small prematures 1500–2500 g	94	89	28	30 %	31%
C. Dysmatures f.t., 1500–2500 g	80	79	29	36 %	37%
D. Large prematures > 2500 g	75	45	15	20 %	33%
E. Full-term >2500 g	1498	260	36	2.4%	14%
Subtotal	1781	489	114	6.4%	23%
II. Extramural	61	42	12	20 %	29%
Total	1842	531	126	6.8%	24%

Table 3. 126 Cases of neonatal hypoglycemia, time of first low glucose-value.

	Cases of hypo-glycemia	0–2 hours after birth	3–6 h.	7–12 h.	13–24 h.	24–48 h.	48–72 h.
A. Very low birth weight	9	7	1	–	1	–	–
B. Small prematures	31	28	–	2	–	1	–
C. Dysmatures	31	20	5	3	1	1	1
D. Large prematures	17	15	–	1	1	–	–
E. Full-term, > 2500 g	38	21	3	5	3	5	1
Total	126	91	9	11	6	7	2

high: 24%, it is still higher in the premature and dysmature groups (34%).
The percentage of hypoglycemia of the total group of newborns (6.8%) is
a minimum for not in every newborn glucose estimations were made.

When we look at the *time* when the first hypoglycemic value was found
it is striking that this happened to be in about a 3/4 of all cases (or 72%)
during the first 2 hours after birth (table 3). It is especially striking in the
groups of premature newborns (groups A, B and D). It applies less clearly
to the dysmature newborns and other full terms.

In many of these cases of early neonatal hypoglycemia we started a
treatment to raise rapidly the glucose values in the blood. The result of
this policy is that we are not well informed about the course blood glucose
values would have taken if we had omitted treatment. In those cases in
which we just observed and checked glucose values regularly we saw that

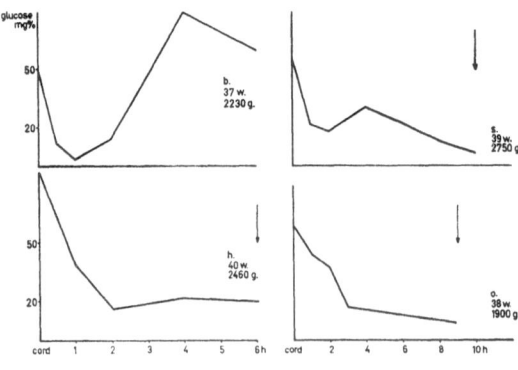

Fig. 1.

one time a rapid increase followed but that at other times an increase of glucose concentration in the blood failed to occur. Sometimes after an initial increase, glucose values may decrease again towards hypoglycemic values (fig. 1).

In the case of an early fall followed by a rapid rise of glucose concentration we are probably dealing with an exaggerated normal physiological dip of the glucose level. Predicting a spontaneous rise from hypoglycemic values is as impossible as predicting a failure of this mechanism, especially in the case of pathological births. This early neonatal hypoglycemia may well be the start of a serious long-term, even symptomatic, hypoglycemia.

When the first hypoglycemic value was found at a later time it relatively often concerned infants that came under 'glucose-control' later.

Considering the *sex* of the newborns with hypoglycemia it is striking to see the preponderance of boys, especially in the low-birth-weight group (table 4). This is a finding consistent with that of other investigators. Still more striking is the preponderance of newborns of *multiparous* mothers in the hypoglycemic group when compared with the normal incidence of multiparity in our clinic. An explanation may be the fact that the occurrence of pathology in multiparous mothers is higher than in primiparous mothers in the admissions to the clinic.

Considering hypoglycemia versus *intra-uterine growth* using the intra-uterine growthcurve in which birthweight is plotted against gestational age, the preponderance of newborns of low-birth-weight for gestational age (or small-for-dates) is very striking (table 5). 70% falls below the

Table 4. Neonatal hypoglycemia versus sex and parity of the mother.

	♂♂	♀♀	Primi	Multi
A. Very low birth weight	3	3	3	3
B. Small prematures	19	9	9	19
C. Dysmatures	17	12	14	15
D. Large prematures	7	8	7	8
E. Full-term, >2500 g	17	19	19	17
Total	63	51	52	62
Total intramural cases of hypoglycemia	55.3%	44.7%	45.6%	54.4%
Total intramural births	53.1%	46.9%	53.4%	46.4%

Table 5. Neonatal hypoglycemia versus intra-uterine growth (according to the intra-uterine growthcurve of Kloosterman and Huidekoper (1969).

	Birthweight percentiles					
	2.3	10	50	90	97.7	
A. Very low birth weight	5	2	2	–	–	–
B. Small prematures	–	2	20	6	–	–
C. Dysmatures	20	6	5	–	–	–
D. Large prematures	–	–	1	11	4	1
E. Full-term, >2500 g	1	10	11	8	2	4
Total	26	20	39	25	6	5
	21%	49%		30%		

50th percentile, 40% below the 10th percentile and more than 20% of all hypoglycemic newborns fall below the 2.3rd percentile which means that their birthweight is more than 2 times the standard deviation below normal for a given gestational age. A correlation between neonatal hypoglycemia and intrauterine growth-retardation is clearly demonstrable. In the group large-for-dates newborns in about 50% infants of diabetic or prediabetic mothers are found.

Considering neonatal hypoglycemia versus some conditions of which is known from earlier studies that they *predispose* toward hypoglycemia it appears that severe dysmaturity as well as toxemia in the mother (which is connected in a distinct way with dysmaturity) occur most frequently (table 6). Neonatal asphyxia also is an important factor linked with hypoglycemia (18%), especially in group E (full-terms, birthweight above 2500 g): ± 30%.

Diabetes and prediabetes occur in all groups of newborns with hypoglycemia. Hypothermia appears to be most important in the smallest newborns, R.D.S. in the group of large prematures.

When we consider, on the other hand, the incidence of hypoglycemia in some 'at risk' groups taken from the total number of newborns it appears again that severe dysmaturity comes in the first place (table 7). In premature infants the incidence is distinctly lower while it increases when we are dealing with the R.D.S.

(Pre)diabetes in the mother and neonatal asphyxia show a distinctly lower incidence of neonatal hypoglycemia. It should be noted however,

Table 6.   126 Cases of hypoglycemia: frequency of predisposing factors.

	A	B	C	D	E	Total
Cases of hypoglycemia	9	31	31	17	38	126
Birthweight below 2.3rd percentile	5	–	20	–	1	26 = 21%
Diabetes or impaired G.T.T. in mother	1	2	6	3	6	18 = 14%
Neonatal asphyxia (Apgarscore 6 or less)	6	1	4	1	11	23 = 18%
Hypothermia (temp. 35°C or less)	5	5	3	–	3	16 = 13%
R.D.S.	4	4	–	8	2	18 = 14%
Toxemia in mother	3	6	9	2	4	24 = 19%

Table 7.   Incidence of neonatal hypoglycemia in some 'at risk' conditions.

	No. of cases	Hypoglycemia	
Birthweight below 2.3rd percentile	59	26 =	44%
Diabetes or impaired G.T.T. in mother	135	17 =	13%
Neonatal asphyxia (group E only) Apgarscore 6 or less	81	11 =	14%
Prematurity	234	55 =	24%
R.D.S. (groups B and D only)	39	12 =	31%
Toxemia in the mother	± 240	22 = ±	9%
Total intramural life-births	1781	114 =	6.4%

that from this survey the number of cases which have been examined for hypoglycemia is not clear. The same holds for toxemia in the mother; the figures suggest a correlation between toxemia in the mother and neonatal hypoglycemia only when there is a coexistent intra-uterine growth retardation.

Hypoglycemia in the smaller one of a very discordant pair of *twins* in which case the smaller one undergoes an intra-uterine growth-retardation, is a very frequent occurrence. In this group were 17 twins with hypoglycemia of which there were 6 pairs of twins with hypoglycemia in both. In 3 further cases it concerned the smaller, in 2 cases the bigger one.

The *treatment* of neonatal hypoglycemia has to consist of supplying

glucose – in severe cases by intra-venous route, in cases that look less
severe by oral route. The trouble is that one cannot always see beforehand
whether one is dealing with a severe case or not. In dysmature newborns
with a distinct hypoglycemia oral glucose supply is insufficient in most
cases, especially in the case of vomiting when feedings do not succeed.

Also in premature infants with respiratory distress the oral glucose
supply is limited.

In the case of full-term newborns with a birthweight of more than
2500 g one will more often meet hypoglycemia of a less serious character,
there will be a greater chance of a spontaneous recovery. Besides, most of
the time oral glucose supply succeeds better in these cases. However in
the case of severe neonatal asphyxia and of infants with a serious, badly-
controlled diabetes in the mother we will sooner use the intra-venous route
for glucose supply.

Considering the total number of newborns with hypoglycemia it appears
that a treatment with intravenous glucose supply was initiated in about
70% of all cases. Of the bigger full term newborns only about 50% was
treated. In general the treatment was started rapidly when the hypoglycemia became known (fig. 2).

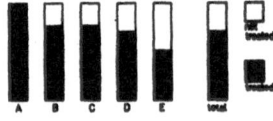

Fig. 2.

When it was decided to treat cases of hypoglycemia which we considered
serious with intravenous glucose supply, an intravenous infusion in a
scalpvein was made by which a glucose-solution of 15% was infused at
a rate of ± 80 ml/kg/24 hours. This accounts for about 8 mg glucose
per kg per minute.

The glucose concentration of the blood has to be checked during the
infusion. The aim is to keep the glucose concentration in the blood above
40 mg%.

If necessary the glucose supply is increased by giving a more concentrated glucose-solution (20%). When the glucose concentration in the
blood rises above 100 mg% it is better to decrease the glucose supply
by giving a less concentrated solution (10% or 5%). Hyperglycemia leads
to hyper-osmolality which is an unfavourable condition.

Oral supply of glucose and formula feeding has to be started as early as possible after birth and should be increased rapidly. When the feedings, given frequently, are tolerated well intravenous supply of glucose may be decreased, while the glucose concentration of the blood is checked regularly.

Intravenous glucose has to be decreased *gradually*. Abrupt stopping may lead to a reactive hypoglycemia – premature stopping may lead to the relapse of a long-lasting hypoglycemia. In the severe cases of neonatal hypoglycemia one has to continue the intravenous glucose supply for about 3–4 days. In part this depends on the quantity of oral feedings given.

I end this paper with some case-reports:
A dysmature newborn with an early neonatal hypoglycemia (fig. 3) treatment with intravenous glucose was started and stopped in the course of the second day. Apparently it was stopped too early. In spite of oral supply a relapse of hypoglycemia occurred on the 4th day.

In another dysmature newborn with early neonatal hypoglycemia (fig. 4) treatment progressed with complications: oral feedings did not succeed at first. While the infusion was running subcutaneously on the first day a relapse of hypoglycemia occurred. In the course of the second day the glucose supply appeared to be insufficient: with a good running infusion a relapse of hypoglycemia occurred again. By increasing the supply the glucose concentration in the blood recovered.

This rather active treatment has the great advantage of preventing long-lasting hypoglycemia and with that symptomatic hypoglycemia. In this group of 126 newborns with neonatal hypoglycemia there was only one

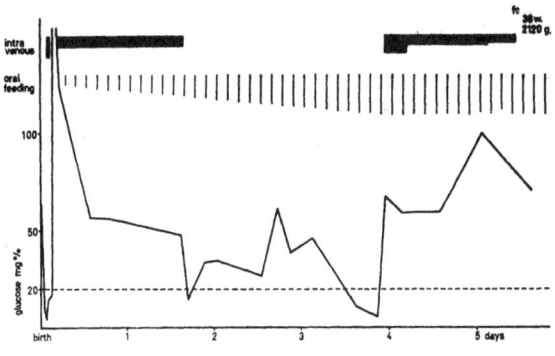

Fig. 3.

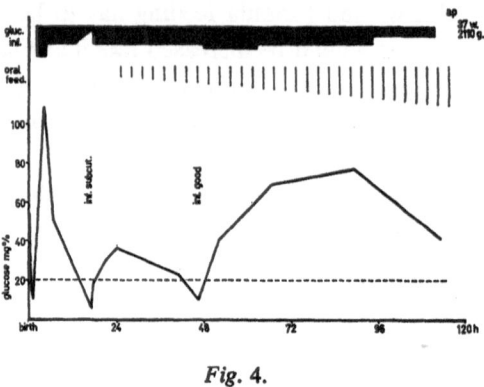

Fig. 4.

case with typical clinical symptoms of hypoglycemia: apnea and convulsions. This newborn (table 8) got no glucose-control from birth. Normal feedings were tolerated well. At the start of the 3rd day convulsions occurred that responded well to intravenous glucose supply. This newborn is the only one of the group that probably did have a long-lasting hypoglycemia and with that will run the real risk of cerebral damage.

   In the cases of symptomatic hypoglycemia it is advised to start treatment with a shot of glucose (a 50% solution): ± 1 g/kg and after that to continue the indicated treatment.

Table 8. A case of symptomatic neonatal hypoglycemia.

Pat. R.W. 2600 grams 37 weeks	Mother epilepsy Pregnancy uneventful Labor uncomplicated Slight asphyxia after birth

Control of bloodglucose was not performed

Feeding from 12 hours after birth (diluted formula with glucose)

	1st day	10 cal/kg	
	2nd day	30 cal/kg	no vomiting

Onset 3rd day:	hypotonia, pallor, apathy, tremors followed by *apnea, cyanosis and convulsions* glucose concentration in the blood: 10 *mg%*

Management:	2.5 g glucose I.V. rapidly infusion glucose 15% 8 mg/kg/min

A rapid improvement followed.

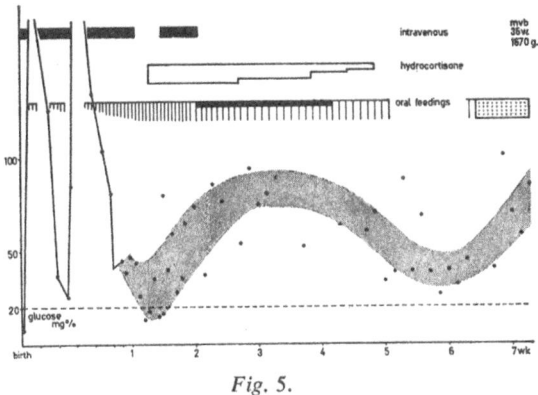

Fig. 5.

In all other cases there were either no symptoms or only aspecific symptoms that occur in other pathological conditions too. Supplying glucose did not correlate with the disappearing of the symptoms in these cases.

Treatment with *corticosteroids* as is advised by some others is not necessary in the great majority of cases. Infusion-therapy is sufficient. In a total of 3 cases (of the 126) we did use corticosteroids. In 2 cases it concerned serious relapsing hypoglycemia. Example:

A premature and dysmature child (fig. 5) that at first caused big problems in regulating the glucose concentration of the blood. After this succeeded and the intravenous glucose supply was stopped, a relapse of hypoglycemia occurred on the 9th day. We then treated with hydrocortison (5 mg/kg/day), another intravenous glucose infusion and addition of glucose to the feedings, later we gave protein-rich feedings. With this regimen a normalisation of the glucose content of the blood was achieved at last. Corticosteroids are used in these cases to stimulate gluconeogenic processes.

Summarizing we can say that neonatal hypoglycemia is a rather frequently occurring condition if we look for it. Its significance, however, is not yet clear. Treatment is easy and is advised in order to prevent possible brain-damage.

REFERENCES

Kloosterman G. J., Over intra-uterine groei en de intra-uterine groeicurve. *Ned. T. Verloskunde* 69, 349 (1969).
Yerushalmy J., The classification of newborn infants by birth weight and gestational age, *J. Pediatr.* 71, 164 (1967).

PANEL DISCUSSION
PART I

MODERATOR A. SIKKEL

Sikkel: Ladies and gentlemen, the papers are open to discussion.

Kubli: Let me first thank you very much for the invitation to come here and for the friendly welcome I have received. Of course I am very sorry to start out with a comment which may reveil some discrepancies between Dr. Gevers and my own present concepts of fetal monitoring. I say present concepts, because certainly these things are going to change.

Dr. Gevers has reported a most interesting study, and I think the only drawback it has is the relatively small number of patients. We are always confronted then with the question whether the sample size is really representative or not. Now, in 900 patients we examined the relationship of the Apgar score of the newborn to the pH in the umbilical artery. With a pH above 7.20 the incidence of Apgar scores of 6 or less was about 5%. In the pH-range between 7.20 and 7.05 we saw 15 to 20% low Apgar scores which means that 80% in this range had a good Apgar score of 7 or more. The incidence of low Apgar scores was 60% at pH-values between 7.05 and 6.95; below 6.95 it was almost 100%. These data mean that undoubtedly a relationship between umbilical artery pH and Apgar scores is present, but that this relationship – except the situation of extreme fetal acidosis – is not a very close one. Now if we do not look at umbilical artery pH, but at fetal capillary blood pH taken at some arbitrarily chosen moment during labour, the relationship of this parameter to clinical depression of the newborn will be even worse *, because labour is a dynamic process during which the biochemical and clinical situation of the fetus may change rapidly. Therefore the accurracy of the prediction of the clinical status of the newborn by means of intrapartum micro blood

---

* Note at the time of correction of manuscripts: In the meantime Hon and collaborators (Obstet. & Gynec., 32, 237, 1969) have clearly demonstrated that the correlation between fetal pH and Apgar score of the newborn is the better the shorter the interval between micro blood sampling and delivery.

sampling certainly is limited. The main problem with micro blood sampling is that this is a discontinuous method and during labour monitoring of the fetus with discontinuous methods is difficult because of the dynamic nature of labour. Undoubtedly clinical results with micro blood sampling will depend largely on the timing and the frequency of sampling in the individual patient.

We have applied micro blood sampling in clinical obstetrics since 1964 and we have not succeeded in substantially lowering intrapartum mortality during labour. It remained the same, at about 4 per thousand until 1967. With the introduction of continuous monitoring of the fetal heart rate it fell to less than one per thousand. Actually this was one fetus out of 1800. This may of course be coincidental but we rather think it is a cause and effect relationship. * We feel that for the prevention of intrapartum death continuous monitoring is better than micro blood sampling, but we fully agree with you that there are discrepancies between the heart rate patterns and the clinical status of the fetus in, I would guess, about 5–10% of the fetuses. I always hope that no one will ask me: Should we do this or should we do that? But personally I prefer continuous monitoring of the fetal heart rate. Of course, if you can, the best thing is to combine both methods, continuous monitoring of FHR *and* micro blood sampling.

Gevers: If I understand you properly, you use both methods in normal and pathological pregnancies. But I believe that in pathological pregnancies the biochemical examination is of much greater value than in the normal cases. Also, it may be that your material was not selected; our material is selected. Another point is that, as you know, when the pH is low during labour, you can better give an oxytocin infusion. Then the pH should improve when the patient is getting pains. This is a factor about which I have not spoken here.

Sikkel: Thank you very much. I think we can start now with the written questions, and perhaps Miss Shelley would be so kind to begin.

Shelley: First question: 'Many years ago, we did not give bicarbonate or glucose to correct acidosis. At least some children survived. How do you account for this survival? Did these children have a high level of glycogen

* During 1969 and 1970 intrapartum mortality stayed at the same low level.

in their tissues as a possible explanation, or are there other explanations?'

I think it likely, on the basis of the data I showed you this morning, that the high glycogen levels in the human foetal heart and liver during the second half of pregnancy were partly responsible. It is likely that this glycogen does have a good deal to contribute towards the survival of the newborn infant. But I think there are other factors, too, besides the amount of glycogen available. Immature tissues do seem to have a greater ability to survive oxygen lack without damage than do adult tissues, and I would like to suggest that this is because the rate of ATP utilization by immature tissues, even when active work is being done, may be lower than that in mature tissues. Studies *in vitro* of the ATP-ase activities of the liver, the brain, and of purified skeletal muscle myosin, have shown that their activity is low in the newborn rat and rabbit and increases towards the adult activity during the first weeks after birth. But in the guinea-pig, which is born in a relatively mature condition with a low ability to survive anoxia, the ATP-ase activities at birth are similar to those in the adult (1, 2, 3, 4, 5, 6). The development of these enzymes is probably associated with an increased capacity for 'work'. For instance, in the brain, the sodium-potassium activated ATP-ase is intimately concerned in the maintenance of the sodium pump and therefore with cerebral activity, and in the skeletal muscles the myosin ATP-ase is essential for muscular contraction. I suspect that in immature tissues the rather low rate of energy production, i.e. of ATP formation, provided by anaerobic glycolysis is sufficient to keep pace with the rate of ATP utilization, so that if you can maintain glycolysis you can prolong survival as in the lambs in mid-gestation. But at a more advanced stage of development, as in foetal lambs and monkeys near term, the rate of ATP utilization is probably faster than earlier in gestation. For instance, just to take one example, the resting blood pressure and the rise in blood pressure in response to oxygen lack are higher in lambs near term than in mid-gestation, suggesting an increase in cardiac work and therefore an increased turnover of ATP in the heart. It is likely that in the lambs and monkeys near term the rate of utilization of ATP was faster than could be sustained by anaerobic glycolysis, the rate of which was similar to that in mid-gestation, and that this was why providing glucose and sodium bicarbonate had little effect on anoxic survival. Thus there are at least two factors involved, the availability of glycogen as a substrate for glycolysis, and the rate of ATP utilization during hypoxia.

This leads to a question put by Dr. Stule. 'In some recent work reported by Assali *et al.* an acid solution was infused into the foetus. No changes in foetal blood pressure or heart rate were observed in these experiments, although the pH dropped below 7.0'.

The important factor in these experiments is probably that there was oxygen available to the foetus. The amount of energy (i.e. ATP) that can be provided by the oxidation of one molecule of glucose all the way to H_2O and CO_2 is something like fifteen times that provided by its anaerobic conversion to lactic acid. So I think that in these experiments, although there may have been some inhibition of glycolysis, the rate of energy production must still have been sufficient to keep the foetus going. There is also a second point to consider. In hypoxia, the source of hydrogen ions is intra-cellular and it is likely that the intracellular pH at the glycolytic site would be affected more than in the experiments cited by Dr. Stule, where the acid was of exogenous origin and may have had little effect on the intra-cellular pH.

Rhemrev: Have you any idea what is the cause of liberation or mobilization of glucose in asphyxiated foetuses? Is it only hypoxia or a low pO_2, or is it due to stress of the foetus?

Shelley: I think there are at least two factors involved here. Comline and Silver (7) have shown in experiments with foetal lambs that asphyxia does cause liberation of catecholamines from the adrenal medulla. In mid-gestation the effect is independent of innervation of the adrenal gland, but near term it is mediated via the splanchnic nerves; if these are cut, there is little liberation of catecholamines in response to asphyxia. But a recent paper (8) has shown that mobilization of glucose can occur in response to splanchnic stimulation even after adrenalectomy of the new-born calf, presumably due to local release of nor-adrenaline within the liver. Both these mechanisms involve catecholamine activation of liver phosphorylase leading to increased glycogenolysis and a rise in blood glucose. But it is also possible that hypoxia may have a direct effect on hepatic glycogen mobilization, for severe hypoxia is likely to cause a rise in the intra-cellular inorganic phosphate and AMP concentrations which will stimulate glycogenolysis quite independently of catecholamine release.

Now there is yet another question: 'What concentration and amount of glucose and base did we use in the anoxic monkeys and lambs?' In these experiments we were monitoring the arterial pH and adjusting the infusion rate to try to keep the pH constant. We used 15% sodium carbonate in

most experiments and a glucose concentration of 10–20%; the mean rate
of infusion in the most successful experiment was about 16 mg sodium
carbonate/kg min. with an equal amount of glucose. But in these experiments the animals were completely anoxic. The amounts necessary in the
clinical situation, where some oxygen is usually available, would probably
be much less.

Drogendijk: You showed a slide concerning the glucose uptake in the
foetus, its oxygen equivalence, and the oxygen consumption, from which
it appeared that about 25% of the glucose is retained unoxidized. Does
this difference correspond to the growth of the foetus or is some other
kind of elimination, such as anaerobic glycolysis, involved?

Shelley: I think the low blood and tissue lactate levels in the normal
foetus suggest that anaerobic glycolysis is no more important in the well-
oxygenated foetus than in the adult. Wolf, Sabata, Frerichs and Melichar
(9) have calculated that in the human foetus the amount of glucose
retained unoxidized is of the right order to account for the amount of fat
and glycogen which accumulates during the latter part of gestation.

REFERENCES TO REMARKS OF H. J. SHELLEY

1. Potter V. R., W. C. Schneider and G. J. Liebl, *Cancer Res.* 5, 21 (1945).
2. Flexner J. B. and L. B. Flexner, *J. cell. Comp. Physiol.* 31, 311 (1948).
3. Herrmann H., J. S. Nicholas and M. E. Vosgian, *Proc. Soc. exp. Biol. Med.* 72, 454 (1949).
4. Dawkins M. J. R., *Proc. R. Soc. B.* 150, 284 (1959).
5. Abdel-Latif A. A. and L. G. Abood, *J. Neurochem.* 11, 9 (1964).
6. Trayer P. and S. V. Perry, *Biochem. Z.* 345, 87 (1966).
7. Comline R. S. and M. Silver, *Br. Med. Bull.* 22, 16 (1966).
8. Edwards A. V. and M. Silver, *J. Physiol. Lond.,* 211, 109 (1970).
9. Wolf, H., V. Sabata, H. Frerichs and V. Melichar. In: Huntingford, P. J., K. A. Hüter and E. Saling, eds., *Perinatal Medicine*, p. 174. Georg Thieme Verlag, Stuttgart (1969).

Stolk: The arterial pO_2 in foetal life is very low by adult standards. Does
it increase gradually to term?

Dawes: The answer is no. The experiments done by other groups using
intra-uterine catheters have shown that it remains approximately constant
during the whole of the latter half of gestation in sheep and monkeys.

Stolk: How did the foetus survive under these conditions?

Dawes: The question is a very interesting one. It survives because there is a very high systemic blood flow to the foetal tissues. This also requires a very large umbilical blood flow.

The systemic blood flow is about three or four times that of the adult. Another question is: Is there a possible compensation mechanism in the maternal blood flow to the placenta, to compensate for increased oxygen utilization by foetus or placenta? Well, this too is an interesting question still unanswered. I know of no investigations on this point, and indeed until the last eighteen months it would have been impossible to design an experiment on this point, because it is only this recently that we have acquired a method for measuring maternal placental blood flow.

Dr. Stolk asks whether I have any data on the effect of changes in maternal blood pH at constant pCO_2 on placental flow, and he draws an analogy between the effects of pH and pCO_2 on simple blood flow. The answer is that this has not yet been studied, again for the same reason, i.e. that it is so recently that we acquired this method for measurement. This is one of the things that has to be investigated. There is some evidence that raising the pCO_2 moderately in the mother does increase the maternal placental blood flow, but I am not entirely satisfied with the results yet.

Van Bemmel: Are alterations in foetal well-being always correlated with changes in foetal blood gas values? Is the change in pCO_2 and pO_2 correlated with changes in foetal circulation and foetal heart action?

Dawes: It is certainly true that changes in pCO_2, pO_2, and pH within the foetus are correlated with changes in foetal circulation and foetal heart action. There is no doubt about that. But I do not know what you would accept nor indeed what I would accept as foetal well-being. How do you measure foetal well-being? Perhaps the best test of any we have yet, is the capacity of the foetus to react to stimuli. We know that if you subject the foetus to quite mild asphyxia, its capacity to respond to central stimuli disappears. It is difficult as yet to give a value as to what pO_2 abolishes this, but I suspect it is of the order of about 10 or 12 mm Hg.

Rhemrev: The better response of the lamb foetus after anaesthesia of the ewe, is that the result of circulation changes due to the pentobarbital?

Dawes: I think this unlikely. It is much more likely to be a direct effect of pentobarbital on brain cells. Dr. Shelley has referred to the fact that immature foetusses in particular have a low ATP-ase level and low utilization of oxygen in the brain, and we do know from other animal experiments done in vitro that pentobarbital reduces the basic metabolic rate of brain cells. This is probably the explanation.

Van Bemmel: What is your opinion about foetal monitoring during birth with respect to prediction of the state of the foetus and foetal distress?

Eskes: I think this is a point Dr. Kubli made quite clear just a few minutes ago. The question is, do we have to monitor at all? Do we have to change our obstetrical attitude? I think a few comments should be made about this. There seems to be a rather silent gap between, let's say, the monitoring people and the clinical people, and perhaps there are a few who are a combination of both. One of the points I want to stress is that the Apgar Score is a semi-quantitative measurement. Before we had these scores we said the baby is doing very well, the baby is doing very bad, or it is in a in between condition; that would mean a score of 8 to 10 or 0 to 2 or in between. I think before we draw any conclusions about monitoring or data acquired during labour, we have to collect just as many concerning the newborn child. And I think that we have not yet arrived at this level. In my opinion, we are gathering data, we are observing labour, as we did before. And in my opinion there is no reason to do very strange things with women on the basis of figures whose basis is still obscure.

I think some of you are familiar with these curves related to labour in the human. The upper channel shows the intra-uterine pressure, the second channel demonstrates the tachogram showing the beat-per-beat integration of the foetal heart, and in the third channel each heart beat of the foetus can be seen. The paper speed is rather slow, because the birth process is very slow. As illustration, figure 1 shows a record of a woman two hours and 12 minutes before delivery. The heart-rate patterns show dips during uterine contractions. When we are 44 minutes before delivery with a dilatation of 8 cm, the foetal heart-rate pattern is unmistakably different from the preceding curve. In this case with ruptured membranes, pH values were within normal limits. Now what does this all mean? Will this child be born healthy or with a low Apgar Score? This is an interesting question. You do not know exactly what happened after this record

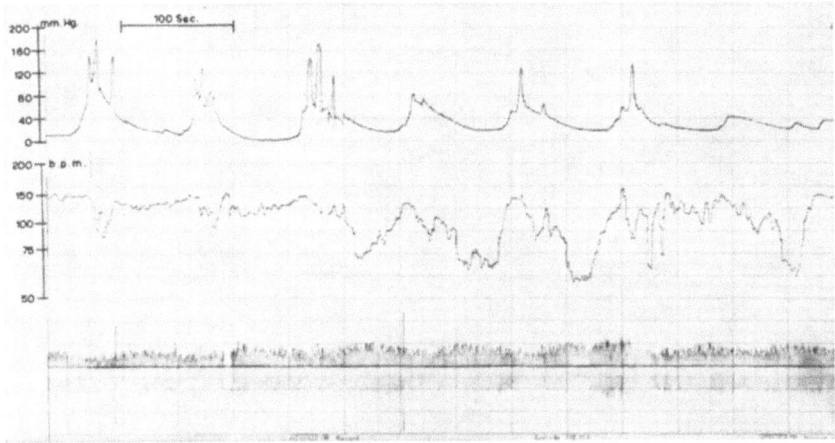

Fig. 1. Record of primigravida, 39 weeks meconiumstained fluid, engaged head. Note the bizar tachogram. pH 7 hrs before birth 7.38, 90 min. before birth 7,27 (after De Haan, Thesis, Vrije Universiteit, Amsterdam 1971).

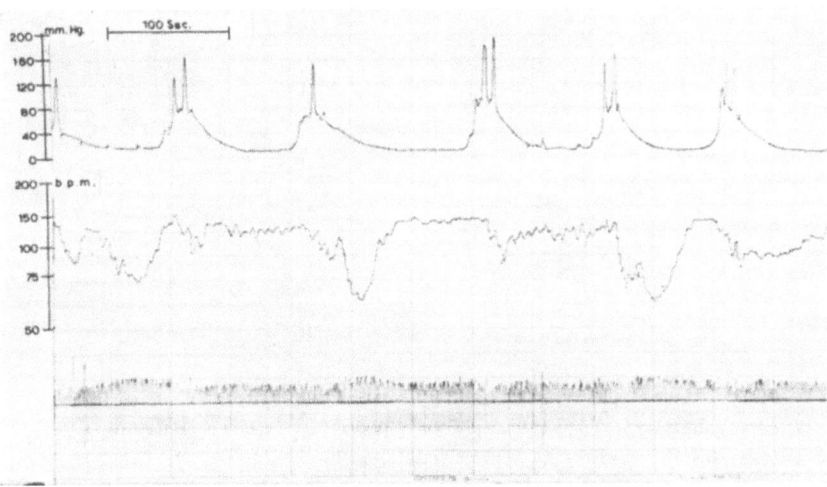

Fig. 2. Continuation of record in figure 1. Actual in this period 7,33. After episiotomy and fundal pressure a boy was born (3530 grams) with an Apgarscore 5 after 2 min. and 7 after 5 minutes. The umbilical cord was twice around the neck (after De Haan, Thesis, Vrije Universiteit, Amsterdam 1971).

was made, and I think no sensible man would dare to guess the answer. Now, this child was born with a very low Apgar Score and the only thing we could see was a very tight encircling of the cord around the neck. The point I want to stress is this. We have looked now for six years at these types of record and we have used miles of paper, but in six years we have not once been able to predict the state of the neonatus all the time. Thanks to our computer, we now can make short-term evaluations of 10 or 15 minutes to tell us exactly in figures what the trend is at, let's say, 11 o'clock, 11.15 and 11.30. And I think we are now at a stage that the computer can give us some help in this prediction, in this so-called foetal trend detection. But I still do not trust the figures, although I like to have lots of them to combine them with classical clinical obstetrics. Perhaps when we have the next course on this subject here in Leiden we will have made progress, and maybe we will be able to show you what figures can mean in foetal evaluation, perhaps even in correlation with the neonatal state. I think I have not answered the question, but I hope I have made something critically clear.

Gevers: May I ask Dr. Eskes how high or low the pH of the umbilical artery was?

Eskes: It was constant at 7.23.

Gevers: That is also the figure we gave. And the Apgar Score was?

Eskes: The Apgar Score was 4.

Gevers: That does not agree with our findings. That Apgar Score is lower than we would expect on the value of the pH of the umbilical artery.

Eskes: That is right.

Sikkel: Thank you very much, Dr. Eskes. I think you have spoken wise words. I agree fully with you that before we draw conclusions from all those figures whose basis we do not know it is extremely important to remember the patient, the woman who is in labour, and to practise clinical obstetrics as we have done for years. I hope that in a few more years we will have more figures and perhaps we will then find that what we are thinking now about the physiology of labour is right, but this is not yet certain. And if you see some patients who are monitored very well and you see that there is no doctor watching the woman herself, I think this may be called a very infortunate situation.

Are there any other questions?

Eskes: I think there is just one remark to make, and that is that the presence of the doctor alone can influence perinatal mortality very much.

Dawes: When the foetal cord lies around the neck and heart beat slows down, is this due to a reduction in the umbilical bloodflow or to venous congestion in the foetal head?

Eskes: That is a very tricky question. I did not look up the answer in your book in time. I think you did not say anything about this point, but we can only speculate about it, because for the human I cannot recall that we have a really good method for measuring foetal bloodflow in the placental or central fetal circulation. If we had such a method, I could answer your question.

Sikkel: You do not get an answer Dr. Dawes. I am very sorry.

Popescu: What do you think about cases of bradycardia in cord compression?

Dawes: I think bradycardia develops in cord compression for two reasons. That is to say, there is a reflex bradycardia because the arterial pressure has gone up. There is no doubt that the baroreceptors work actively quite early in foetal life in those species that have been investigated. Certainly they are working very well immediately after birth. But it is also true that even if the vagus is cut, you can still get bradycardia during asphyxia. There is a direct effect upon the heart, when pO_2 is reduced below 10 mm Hg. This bradycardia in the human infant during delivery, in circumstances where clear evidence is obtained at delivery or from micro-blood samples showing that the foetus is hypoxic, is extremely interesting. Because it means that the ordinary mechanisms of foetal blood gas homeostasis have been overwhelmed. It is certainly an extreme degree of oxygen lack that can produce this form of bradycardia in the foetus. The baroreceptors are located in the aortic arch and in the carotid sinus. In the adult, the pulmonary arterial receptors and the ventricular receptors have been investigated extensively, but we know practically nothing about their function in foetal life. There are just too few investigators in this field.

Sikkel: Here is another question for the team of Dr. Gevers. The question is: 'you showed an illustration with an extremely low pH value in the umbilical artery and an extremely high glucose content. But that was not the same patient. Is there in every case a correlation between a low pH and a high glucose content?' Perhaps Dr. Rhemrev can answer this question.

Rhemrev: It should be, but we have not found it!

Sikkel: Here is a last question for the team of Dr. Gevers. Was there also a lowering of perinatal mortality and of the frequency of caesarean sections during the period in which perinatal monitoring was applied?

Gevers: Yes, there was a lowering of our perinatal mortality and a drop in the frequency of caesarean sections.

MODERATOR F. KUBLI

Kubli: Ladies and gentlemen, we have quite a lot of questions. There are a few addressed to myself, and if you don't mind I shall start with them, so we can finish with the foetus and the main topic of this session. There is a question from Dr. Gevers, who would like to discuss his results on oxytocin infusion.

Gevers: We have asked ourselves whether the oxytocin infusion itself contributed to an intensification of the pathology or not, or was the effect due solely to the pathological condition itself. I will show you the results of our experiments.

Normal group

with oxytocin inf.	without oxytocin inf.
5 cases	12 cases
mean pH umb. art. 7.24	mean pH umb. art. 7.26

Pathological group

with oxytocin inf.	without oxytocin inf.
12 cases	4 cases
mean pH umb. art. 7.175	mean pH umb. art. 7.10
	(without the lowest value: 7.19)

For the normal group, with oxytocin infusion there were only 5 cases of prolonged labour. The mean pH of the umbilical artery was 7.24. Without oxytocin infusion there were 12 cases; the mean pH of the umbilical artery was 7.26. Thus, the difference is lower than in your figures.

In the pathological group there were 12 cases with oxytocin infusion because there was pathology. The mean pH of the umbilical artery was 7.175. Without oxytocin infusion there were 4 cases; the mean pH of the umbilical artery was 7.10. If the very low pH of 6.82 is not taken into account, the mean value becomes 7.19. It is clear that there is also no real difference between these figures. The explanation is perhaps that we set the dosage of the oxytocin infusion somewhat lower. We give two units per 500 ml, and in some instances only one unit. When we see on the recordings of the intra-uterine pressure that the pressure is too high, we place the patient on her left or right side, after which we often see that the high basal tone or the high peaks diminish. That is a possible explanation.

Kubli: I fully agree. What I am trying to make clear is that it is not a matter of oxytocin alone. It is a matter of dosage, of the method of administration and of proper control. What we were struck by was the fact that before monitoring we had not been aware of how bad our oxytocin administration was. I would certainly admit that you can do better. I think the same problem is involved in a question put by Dr. Eskes. He says: 'It seems to me, in comparison with our recently published studies on oxytocin stimulation that 49% of abnormal uterine activity in the oxytocin group is very high. Could it be that this is due to the method of administration in which more oxytocin is given than you think?'

Yes, I think that might be the case, although I must stress that we had observed as much as 17% hyperactivity during spontaneous labour without oxytocin. Dr. Eskes has brought up another interesting point. He felt that patients with postmaturity, toxemia, meconium stained amniotic fluid etc. were especially inclined to develop abnormal uterine activities. I do not have precise results of my own, but I think – and this is just an impression – that this might be correct. This would mean that patients with 'placental insufficiency' are especially prone to have unco-ordinated and with that also hyperactive labour. Our own results certainly would have to be discussed with respect to this possibility: The oxytocin group including more patients with signs of placental insufficiency than the control group, the increased incidence of uterine hyperactivity might in part be due to the selection of the patients. I think we all agree that the problem of uterine hyperactivity is not solved by simply condemning oxytocin. We were struck by some very queer things we saw, e.g. the effect of bladder voiding during spontaneous labour.

At the moment of spontaneous bladder voiding or catheterization you may see a perfect uterine hypertonus without any oxytocin. Vaginal manipulation also may cause uterine hyperactivity. So I think there is quite a lot still to be studied.

Gevers to Spierdijk: Do you make a distinction between primary and secondary caesarean sections? In how many cases were primary caesarean sections performed and what were the results?

Spierdijk: Most of the cases were primary caesarean sections: only in two cases of pre-eclampsia were secondary caesarean sections concerned, and those were dysmature babies with low Apgar Scores. In our hospital it was difficult to collect data at night and during week-ends.

Gevers: Why did you not take blood from the umbilical artery? That would have given you more reliable information.

Spierdijk: I agree, but I started this investigation before I became aware of Eckenhausen's investigations. If I were to start such a study now, I would sample the blood in the umbilical artery.

Gevers: I think the metabolic acidosis in the mother is not the result of hyperventilation but of fasting during labour. Did you see hyperventilation and for how long?

Spierdijk: After at least six hours of hyperventilation there is a possibility of renal compensation. Among the patients with normal Apgar Scores, there was one hyperventilating mother. Among these 33 patients there was only one woman with a very low pCO_2 value, and that was 16.5. We did not see a decrease in the Apgar Score, but I think the hyperventilation was not of long duration.

Gevers: Hyperventilation during labour usually occurs in a period during the last hours, in the second stage.
   Hyperventilation does not develop in the beginning of labour, but fasting during labour occurs during a much longer period. We have seen the results of fasting: when the mother is given glucose you can see recovery in the values of micro-blood examination in the child.

Spierdijk: That was the reason why I started to observe the pH. When we have a prolonged period of acidity there must have been a primary hyperventilation. But when the period is limited, we are dealing with primary metabolic acidosis. I think that when the mother is nervous and upset before labour had gone on very long and she has been taken to the hospital, she is possibly hyperventilating. And there was no question of labour at the time. I hope to pursue this investigation further in patients who are upset before operations.

Popescu: Dr. de Leeuw asks: 'Can we have some information about promazin?' Yes, the studies on promazin were published by Selwyn Crawford in 1965 in the British Journal of Anaesthesia.

We have to take into account the influence of pregnancy but also, according to newer studies (1966), the influence of oral contraceptives who both slow the metabolism of promazin.

The initial well controlled study was performed on 15 patients receiving in groups of 5 a standard dose of 50 mg either intramuscularly, intravenously, direct or in infusion. Concentration of promazin and total amount of it and two of its metabolites were determined in the urine of neonates. Figure 8 must be remembered: it is clear that with intravenously administered drug to the mother concentration as well as the total amount of drug excreted by the neonate is much higher (concentration ± 5 times, total amount ± 3 times higher). But it is even more interesting to note that concentrated intravenous administration in the mother gives rise to the highest concentration in neonatal urine while intravenous infusion of the same quantity produces a lower concentration of eliminated drug in the neonate but a larger total amount of elimination. This is a demonstration of the role that the two factors: high blood concentration in the mother (direct intravenous injection) and time (infusion method), are playing in placental transfer. There are factors of error in this study:

The weight of the parturients was not equal although the dose was standard (50 mg) and also the time of administration before partus couldn't be the same because of the unpredictable moment of birth, but the data are highly suggestive.

Kubli: Thank you very much Dr. Popescu. If there are no other questions for Dr. Popescu, we can proceed to the newborn. Dr. Ruys will read the questions.

Ruys: Thank you very much, Mr. Chairman. The first question, from Dr. van Ek, is as follows: 'Should I conclude from your lecture that prematures with a respiratory distress syndrome have a birth weight that is in accordance with their gestational age? In other words: do small prematurely born children show the respiratory distress syndrome in a higher number of cases?' I will answer this question by saying that it is my impression that the respiratory distress syndrome is correlated much more clearly with gestational age than with birth weight. In cases in which R.D.S. was not correlated with low gestational age but occured in small for dates babies, I have seen several times that other abnormalities, such as congenital malformations of the heart, were present.

Then there are two questions, one from Professor de Bruyne and one from Dr. Steenhuizen, asking why we in Leiden no longer use a THAM solution for the correction of acidosis. My first remark is that series in the literature indicate that the neonatal mortality rate is not differently affected by the use of sodium bicarbonate for the correction of acidosis or by the use of a THAM solution. Moreover, sodium bicarbonate offers the advantage that we can use a smaller volume, three times as small as when we use Tris buffer. In addition, the supposed advantage of the THAM solution, i.e. that it decreases the pCO_2, is only an effect of very short duration, and gives rise, as I have already said in my paper, to a lowering of the respiratory stimulation. If you see more lowering of pCO_2, I think this is an effect not of Tris itself but rather of a better pulmonary circulation. And this is the same effect we see after the use of sodium bicarbonate. So, in my opinion, a Tris buffer has no advantage over the use of sodium bicarbonate.

Kubli: Dr. Ruys, could you comment on the problem of an intracellular action of THAM or against bicarbonate?

Ruys: I know from the literature that the intracellular action of THAM has been mentioned as an advantage, but it may be that this action does not exist at all (Irvine et al. 1966, Metabolism, *15*, 1011); but perhaps Dr. Dawes can comment on this problem.

Kubli: Dr. Dawes, would you like to comment?

Dawes: From a clinical point of view, I would say that if THAM solution can possibly inhibit respiration, it should be omitted. When large amounts of sodium bicarbonate are used, you have to watch the serum sodium level.

Ruys: Yes, I fully agree. I did not see an important elevation of the sodium level, but, as I have already told you, I was impressed by a rather marked lowering of the serum protein level due to the dilution of the blood by the hypertonic solution. And that brings me to the following question from Dr. van Aken. He wants to know what kind of doses I apply. We are using the formula of Dr. Hutchison: BE x kg body weight x 0.35 = $NaHCO_3$ in meq. The amount of sodium bicarbonate in meq. is the same as the amount in ml when you use the 8.4 percent concentration. The next question is whether I am inclined to give this amount directly or in several portions. Usually we give two-thirds of this amount of sodium bicarbonate at once, as fast as possible. But since I noticed this drop in serum protein level during the last few months, I am inclined, if I have to use a rather large amount of sodium bicarbonate, to give one-half of the total amount directly and the second part by drip infusion for example.

Dr. van der Meulen asks whether the use of the Dräger pulmotor is more reliable than mouth-to-mouth ventilation. I think the pulmotor has the advantage that it can be used in the incubator without opening the hood and therefore avoids the risk of further cooling of the infant. Moreover, it is an instrument that can be used by even a rather inexperienced nurse, whereas the mouth-to-mouth ventilation demands a little more experience and may be more effective for a longer time than the use of the pulmotor, because, although you may want so, you cannot change the inspiratory volume of the pulmotor.

The last question asks: What it the incidence of organic brain damage in children when acidosis persists in spite of corrective measures? And is secondary artificial ventilation justified in view of the future of these children? This is a subject we could discuss for several hours, I suppose, and it is also the subject of the Saturday morning session. I think we shall have time for it in the panel discussion. I can make one remark now: for a child with a persisting acidosis and no evidence of an intracranial haemorrhage, which we can confirm roughly with a lumbar puncture, I think that artificial ventilation of longer duration is indicated.

Kubli: Thank you very much Dr. Ruys. May I comment briefly on your last words? I have been impressed by a small study published in the Proceedings of the last Ross Conference, concerning cerebral damage, showing that for long-term artificial respiration in prematures having apnoea due to immaturity, there is a relatively good prognosis in terms of cerebral damage, whereas babies born in hypoxia and having had asphyxia at birth, had a relatively poor prognosis. I have one question to put to Dr. Ruys. Did I understand you correctly, that you correct acidosis in all babies that have a pH in the umbilical artery below 7.20? Is that correct? We found a pH of less than 7.20 in about one-third of all the babies born in our department, and in about 20 percent of the babies that were clinical normal in all respects. So this would mean one out of five absolutely normal babies. Could you comment on that?

Ruys: Yes, as I have already told you, an estimation of the pH value and derived values is only done (if no estimation has been performed during labour) after delivery of a child with an Apgar Score of 7 or less or with a low birth weight. So we have first of all a child with an Apgar Score of 7 or less, and if the pH is lower than 7.20, then in my opinion there is an indication for correction of the acidosis.

Kubli: Thank you. Can the panel advise us about parameters to be used in a non-academic hospital for the adequate care of the newborn and especially the prematures? What is, for instance, the value of lactate determination? I think that this is an important question, because we keep talking about it but most of the people here are not working in a university hospital. Perhaps you can very briefly give some advise as to what to do when an Astrup apparatus is not available, whether you can correct blindly, and what you would advise. I think that might be interesting for the audience.

Ruys: If you have a child with a low Apgar Score, let us say 7 or less, you can administer sodium bicarbonate without making an estimation of pH and of derived values, and you can administer 3 meq. per kg body weight. This corresponds to a base excess of –10 meq. in a full-term infant. I think that you can do this without danger of overcorrection, and you can repeat it, if the child is in a bad condition, after one hour. But I think that before you repeat this correction you should have an estimation of the infant's pH.

Kubli: Thank you very much. Dr. de Leeuw, will you discuss a question from Dr. Smith: Have you had any experience with the initial treatment of hypoglycaemia with glucagon?

De Leeuw: I can tell you our experience with infants of diabetic mothers with hypoglycaemia. We have sometimes seen a good response of the glucose level, but the effect of glucagon is not reliable. If check estimations are done, a drop in the glucose level is often found after an initial rise. So you have to give an infusion in these cases too. Theoretically, it is perhaps not wise to use glucagon in infants of diabetic mothers, for it has been known for some years that glucagon promotes insulin release, which is unfavourable in view of the hyper-insulinism in these infants. We have had some experience with the use of glucagon in dysmature infants. We saw a rise but sometimes only a very small rise that was followed by a decrease.

Gevers: In the group of term babies, a distinction was made between 'good' babies and 'bad' babies? If so, what kind of criteria did you use?

De Leeuw: I set the limit at an Apgar Score of 6 or less. Among the series of 38 term babies of normal birth weight with neonatal hypoglycaemia, there were 11 cases of asphyxia.

Kubli: I have a question of my own. If you have a baby like this, how often do you have to check blood glucose to be sure not to miss the substantial period of hypoglycaemia? This is of great practical importance.

De Leeuw: We do the estimation every hour during the first hours after birth; we estimate the glucose value in the mixed cord blood, after one hour and after two hours, and when the glucose level is below 20 mg percent one hour after birth and there is a spontaneous rise above 20 mg percent two hours after birth, we just observe further and check glucose values regularly.

Popescu: What does regular mean?

De Leeuw: The frequency of the estimation depends on the values we find. But in practice it is often so that in cases occurring at the end of the evening we start earlier with an infusion therapy than during the day.

Kubli: Can you give a little more detail? You perform an estimation hourly during the first two hours and then if the value remains at about 30 or 40 mg percent, you do it every three hours, to give a rough schedule?

De Leeuw: Yes, even when a child is born at night it is not so difficult to see whether it has a low glucose level. When there is no technician available who can determine it exactly, you can use the dextro-sticks to estimate the glucose level. The result is not quite exact, but you can see whether the level is low or normal. Our experience with the dextro-stick estimation is that it is not reliable for values below 40 mg percent; we get many false – negative and false – positive results. Besides it is impossible for the resident to do the dextro-stick estimations all night, but I suppose that it is not so bad when it happens that you give one glucose infusion too much.

Kubli: Thank you. Are there any more questions?

Reepmaker: Dr. Ruys has not answered my question fully, because I should like to know what parameters you advise to be used in the care of the child, and especially what is the value of the lactate determination in the blood?

Ruys: The lactate determinations have the disadvantage that normally you have to use a rather large amount of blood. It is only for the last few months that we have applied the micro-determination in our Obstetric Department, and I have no experience in the use of lactate as a parameter for treatment of the infant. As I have already stressed, I am inclined to think that there are two or three indications for bicarbonate treatment: a low Apgar Score, especially when combined with acidosis (if you have the equipment to do that determination) and cases of children with a low birth weight who are also born with a low Apgar Score. But it is difficult to give other parameters. If you cannot do an Astrup determination you must watch the clinical condition and check whether the child looks better after treatment with sodium bicarbonate.

Kubli: Thank you very much. May I just add that to my simple mind a lactate determination has no place in practical management, because it takes too long. I think that the base excess value serves the purpose adequately. Lactate is a beautiful research parameter but is not suitable for practical application.

COMPARISON OF VENTILATORS FOR NEWBORNS AND PREMATURES

D. H. G. KEUSKAMP

It hardly to be said that for the ventilation of premature and newborn infants the characteristics of the ventilation are chosen on the basis of physiological values with respect to tidal volume and frequency, and that the positive pressures developing during this ventilation must be kept below a certain limit.

The tidal volume of a newborn amounts on the average to 15 ml and of a prematurely born child even to between 5 and 12 ml. The respiratory frequency amounting to about 45 per minute in a healthy infant can reach as much as 60 per minute in prematures.

In the ventilation of healthy infants pressures occur that are not higher than those seen in the ventilation of adults. Although the compliance (of thorax + lungs) is smaller in infants than in adults, the same holds for the tidal volume, so that the pressure is of the same order of magnitude: between 5 and 10 cm H_2O.

When there is an indication for ventilation, however, an unfavourable situation must be taken into account in which the compliance is markedly reduced (in atelectasis, the respiratory distress syndrome, after extensive intra-abdominal surgery, etc.), which requires adaptation of the ventilation: limited compliance means that a higher pressure is needed to reach the same tidal volume in the lungs. This pressure can reach dangerously high values, even up to 50 cm H_2O, which can lead to such complications as pneumothorax, mediastinal emphysema, pneumopericardium, and subcutaneous emphysema, quite apart from the unfavourable influence on the pulmonary bloodflow.

In such cases the only alternative is to reduce the tidal volume and to increase the frequency of ventilation to reach the required minute volume. A higher frequency means a shortening of the respiratory cycle: at a frequency of 60 per minute a cycle lasts 1 second. At a ratio of 1 : 1 for the inspiration and expiration phase, inhalation lasts half a second, at a ratio of 1 : 2 even one-third of a second.

When even a small tidal volume must be brought into the lung within such a short time, however, a relatively high 'peak pressure' develops and the inflowing gas cannot distribute itself adequately over lung regions with mutually divergent compliance: the gas will take the path of least resistance, resulting in an uneven irregulary ventilation-perfusion ratio. This creates a dilemma between a long inspiratory phase – with a better distribution of the gas in regions with poor compliance but with a longer duration of positive pressure having a disadvantageous influence on the pulmonary circulation – and a shorter inspiratory phase with a lighter load on the pulmonary circulation but with a high peak pressure and unequal gas distribution.

The proper ratio between inspiration and expiration cannot be predicted and varies from case to case, even from time to time in the same infant. Therefore, there must be a simple means to modify this I : E ratio, so that the ventilation pattern can be continuously adjusted to changing conditions. The compliance can change repeatedly in correspondence with the development or disappearance of atelectasis, the filling of the child's stomach, or changes in the position of the baby. It is therefore important for the ventilation apparatus to be what is called volume constant, i.e. the delivered tidal volume must not be dependent on the pressure developed, in contrast to the so-called pressure cycled machines in which the pressure is constant but therefore the tidal volume variable (fig. 1).

On the basis of these considerations a number of criteria can be formulated that a ventilator for use with newborns and premature babies must satisfy:

1. The frequency must be adjustable over a range of from 20 to 80 per minute.
2. The inspiration to expiration ratio must be adjustable from 1 : 1 to 1 : 3.
3. The tidal volume must be adjustable to values from 5 to 100 ml.
4. The tidal volume must be constant and independent of changes in the compliance or the resistance in the air passages.
5. It must be possible to warm and humidify the gaseous mixture such that it reaches the lungs at a temperature of about 35°C ($\pm$ 2°C) and a relative humidity of at least 75 per cent.

The following features are desirable in a ventilator:

a. The possibility of negative pressure during the expiratory phase.

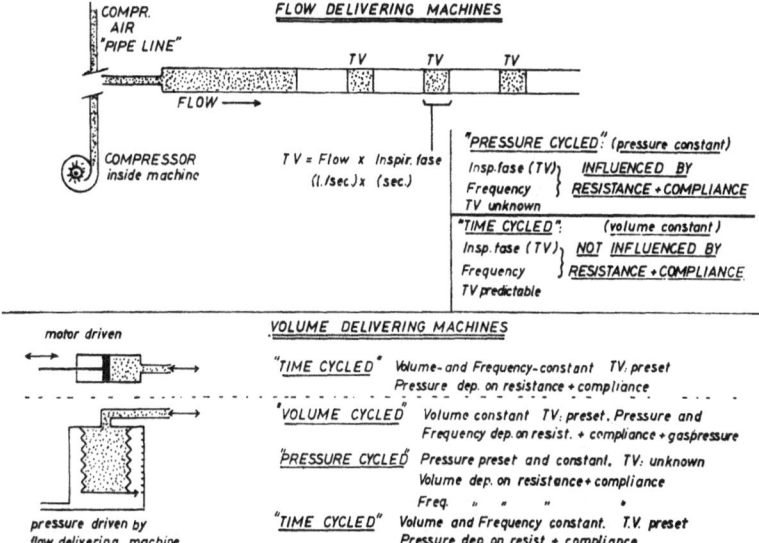

Fig. 1. Schematic classification of ventilation machines according to their characteristics.

Flow-delivering machines: a constant but adjustable gas flow is divided into 'portions'. The size of the portion (the tidal volume) is determined by the duration of the inspiratory phase, which in turn is determined by: the pre-set ventilation pressure (pressure cycled): the delivered volume and often the frequency as well are then dependent on compliance and resistance; or the pre-set inspiration time (time cycled): the delivered volume is not dependent on compliance and resistance, but the pressure rises as the compliance decreases and the resistance increases.

Volume-delivering machines: These supply a given pre-adjustable volume, either by a mechanically-driven pump or by a harmonica bellows operated mechanically or by air pressure. In the former case the frequency is determined by the number of revolutions of the motor and the volume to be supplied is regulated by the stroke of the piston. In the latter case the volume is determined by the excursion of the bellows, the frequency and pressure being dependent on the adjustment of the pneumatic drive mechanism.

b. The possibility of a slight positive pressure during the expiratory phase.

c. Small dimensions of the apparatus.

d. Easy and convenient operation of the apparatus.

e. The breathing tubes should not hamper nursing and manipulation of the infant in the incubator more than absolutely necessary.

Elucidation of points 1–5 and a–e

1 and 2: The argumentation concerning these points has already been given above.

3: The small tidal volume must be adjustable and known. This criterion is not satisfied by any ventilator constructed for adults, because the internal volume (internal compliance or internal compressible dead space) of these machines is too large; consequently, during the inspiratory phase this volume – often several liters – is compressed and there is no longer any relationship between the predicted and delivered volume (See fig. 2).

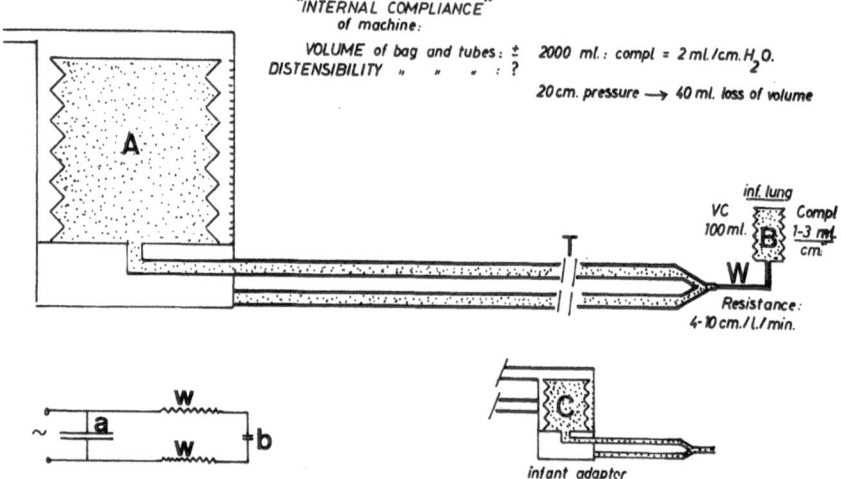

Fig. 2. 'Internal Compliance'. The large harmonica bellows (A) ventilates the infant lung (B) in this schematic representation. These two compartments form a single compressible volume, but are separated by the resistance (W) At higher frequencies and small respiratory volumes, the machine compresses mainly its 'own' volume. An electronic analog elucidates the 'levelling' effect of this situation on the small pressure variations the respiratory volume must convey to the infant's lungs: the delivered volume is much lower than the pre-set volume. Insertion of a small harmonica bellows (C) at T makes no change in this situation except that the delivered volume can now be read more accurately.

4: The compliance can change continuously, as already mentioned, but this also holds for the resistance in the very narrow endotracheal tube, in which mucus or torsion can diminish the size of the lumen.

5: Adequate warning and humidification of the air supply is imperative to prevent drying out of mucus in the air passage and tube. The temperature of the inspired gas must be controlled (not higher than 37°C), and humidification must be achieved by saturation with water vapour, not by a mist technique. With the latter method the child receives indeterminable quantities of distilled water, which can lead to a disturbance of the electrolyte balance; and, furthermore, it is not certain that the droplets will penetrate as far as the smallest air passages, which means that these droplets can contribute to the relative humidity only by evaporation. Lastly, the administration of such a mist requires tubes of a relatively large diameter if precipitation of the droplets is to be avoided.

a: For the ventilation of infants, narrow tubes – with an internal diameter of up to 2.5 mm – are introduced into the tranchea. The resistance of these tubes to the airflow is great, and demands a ventilation pressure considerably higher than the pressure in the lung. During the inspiratory phase this is not objectionable, because the machine can overcome this resistance, but it hampers expiration, which occurs passively, even to the extent that after a few breaths a positive pressure is built up in the lungs, since they cannot empty before a new inspiration begins. This complication can be avoided by applying a slight negative pressure – corresponding to the resistance of the tube – during the expiration phase. But under no condition may a negative pressure develop in the lung.

b: A positive pressure in the lungs after the inspiratory phase – resulting from the resistance described under point a – can be useful in cases of atelectasis and the respiratory distress syndrome, because it can contribute to the gradual expansion of poorly aerated parts of the lungs, and it may also be assumed that the passage of fluid from the lung capillaries to the alveolar space is impeded by the positive pressure in a way comparable to the effect of positive-pressure ventilation in cases of pulmonary oedema.

c: Small dimensions of the apparatus seems to be a superfluous restriction, but experience has shown that the available space around an incubator in a hospital department for prematures and newborns, and certainly in isolation rooms, is apparently determined according to the size of the patients. A large ventilation machine limits the accessibility of the incubator for the nurse and the physician and means that the ventilation tubes must be unnecessarily and harmfully long.

d: Simplicity of operation is an essential condition. In practice, ventilation is performed by the nursing staff under the advice and instruction of the physician. The operation of the apparatus must be easy to understand and the number of possible adjustments must be restricted to the most essential. The more knobs there are the greater the chance of errors and misunderstandings.

e: Even under uncomplicated circumstances a premature infant is difficult to maintain in an incubator, when chilling, infection, and disturbance of an intravenous infusion must be avoided. When a ventilation tube is used, it must remain possible to manipulate and move the child. This can only be done if the ventilation tube is thin and flexible, so that the head does not have to be fixed in one position.

In recent years the variety of ventilation apparatus available has increased greatly, and it has already become difficult for the physician to make a choice, since he cannot evaluate them on a comparative basis. For this reason, the Internation Organization for Standardization IOS appointed a committee to design a 'test program' for ventilation equipment that would show all the characteristics of the apparatus and permit comparison of these characteristics and the performance with those of other machines.

In these tests the ventilation apparatus is subjected to a load comparable to that occurring at the ventilation of a patient. The tests are based on several selected values for the tidal volume, frequency, and inspiration-to-expiration ratio, the values being related to the age of the patient according to three groups: adults, children, and infants.

The load is formed by:

a. The reducing of the 'compliance' of the lung model.
b. The increasing of the resistance in the air passages.

a. The lung model consists of a container with rigid walls whose volume determines the 'compliance'. A 50-litre container simulates a (linear) compliance of 50 ml/cm H_2O pressure. Containers of 50, 30, 20, 10, 3, and 1 litre volume simulate the compliance of adults to premature infants. The containers are heat-insulated and are provided with a large quantity of copper gauze (from 10 to 0.5 kg) to avoid adiabatic compression.

b. The resistances in the air passage are simulated by resistances that must be linear with the air flow over a range of 1 litre/min to 1 litre/sec. The resistance values are taken at 5, 20, 50, 200, and 500 cm H_2O per 0,5 litre/sec.

Since within the scope of the present report we are concerned with the machines suitable for the ventilation of newborn and premature infants, only the following test situation will be discussed:

a. Compliance of 3 ml/cm H_2O and 1 ml/cm H_2O, corresponding to containers with a volume of 3000 and 1000 ml, respectively.
b. Resistances of 5, 20, 50, 200, and 500 cm H_2O per 0,5 litre/sec.

For the sake of clarification it should be mentioned that high resistances in the presence of a small gas flow, such as occur in the ventilation of infants (0.5 to 2 litre/min) give a real resistance of the order of 10 to 50 cm H_2O. Such pressures indeed occur during the ventilation of infants with the hyaline membrane syndrome and where small endotracheal tubes are used.

Fig. 3 gives a schematic representation of the test design and the resulting curves. The resistance R simulates a resistance in the air passage. EP (extrapulmonary pressure) is the pressure measured at the entrance to the air passage, IP (intrapulmonary pressure) is the pressure in the lung. The difference between EP and IP, shown by the superimposed curves, EP/IP, is the pressure loss over the resistance R. The curve FL gives the gas flow in litres/minute, and this value integrated over the inspiration time is a measure of the tidal volume TV. The gas flow is measured by means of a differential pressure transducer and a Fleisch pneumatograph. Compartments C1 and C3 represent the containers with a 'compliance' of 1 ml/cm H_2O and 3 ml/cm H_2O, respectively.

The schematically indicated curves given here originate from the graphs obtained from the tests run on various ventilation machines. As examples of the tests only the results for a few types widely used in The Nether-

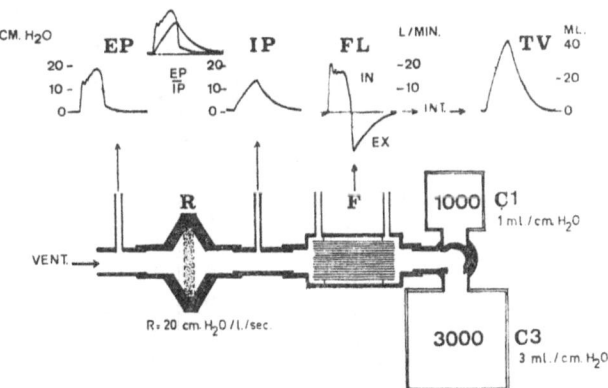

Fig. 3. Schematic representation of the test design. The ventilator is attached at the point VENT. EP: the pressure supplied by the ventilator, i.e. the ventilation pressure. IP: the pressure in the lungs. R: the resistance in the air passage. F: Fleisch pneumotachograph. Fl: air flow at inspiration (IN) and expiration (EX). TV: the tidal volume. C1 and C3: the compartments, having a compliance of 1 ml/cm H_2O and 3 ml/cm H_2O, respectively.

lands can be given. In the test set-up only the resistance is varied, the 'compliance' being kept constant.

The concept 'internal compliance of the ventilator' is elucidated in Fig. 2 on the basis of the large machines constructed for adults in which a given tidal volume is supplied by a pump or bellows. The latter can be operated mechanically or by air pressure. The machine's 'own' volume usually amounts to several litres, in contrast to the vital capacity of an infant lung of about 0.1 litre. The pressure increase in the combined internal area (machine + patient) compresses mainly the air in the machine (internal compressible dead space), which means that the relationship between the supplied and delivered tidal volume is incertain, with increasing divergence as soon as a resistance makes higher ventilation pressures necessary.

From the following graphs the 'characteristics' of the ventilator are clearly evident. They show the extent to which the supplied tidal volume becomes modified with increasing ventilation pressure, the extent to which the frequency remains constant, whether the machine is pressure constant or volume constant, etc.

These characteristics tell little about the quality of the apparatus and only how much the performance is in agreement with the wishes of the practitioner – in this case for the ventilation of infants.

◄ : on demand

	FREQ 60	TV 5	VOL. CONST	FREQ CONST	PRESS CONST	TV predict	Int Com SMALL	Neg.Pr.	I.E Ratio variable	SIMPL control	EASY handling	SMALL SIZE
Engstrom				●			●					
Spiromet + appl.	●	●		●	◄		●	●				
BLease				●			●	●				
Cape				●			●			●		
Bird	●	●			●		●	●	●			●
Bennett	●	●			●		●	●	●			●
Bird + appl.	●	●	◄		◄		●	●			●	●
Aga	●	●			●		●			●		
Airshields	●				●		●			●		
Barnett II				●	◄	●		●	●			
Amst. Inf. Vent.	●	●	●	●	◄	●	●	●	●	●	●	●
Sheffield	●	●	●	●	●	●	●		●	●	●	●
Bourns	●	●	●	●	◄	●	●			●		

Fig. 4. Characteristics of several ventilation machines tested on the basis of the discussed lung model and with respect to the criteria stipulated in the present paper.

SOME EXAMPLES OF VENTILATOR CHARACTERISTICS

For these examples the machine was set for a frequency of 60/min and a tidal volume of 30 ml. Compliance amounted to 1 ml/cm H_2O. For each run the respiration resistance was raised from 0 to 20, 50, 200, and 500 cm $H_2O/0.5$ litre/second. With this load no change is made in the adjustment of the ventilator.

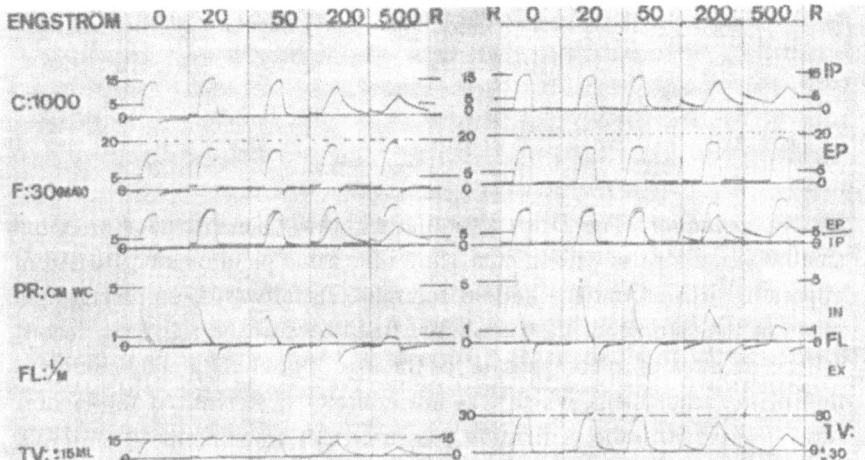

Engström ventilator: The maximal frequency of the Engström ventilator is 30/min. At a load of R 200, it can be seen that for an pre-set tidal volume of both 15 ml and 30 ml this decreases and with R 500 drops to half the pre-set value. The IP (pressure *in* the lung) no longer drops to zero when the load is R 200 and R 500: the lungs no longer empty (trapping), which makes the application of a negative pressure during the expiration phase desirable. For this otherwise volume-constant ventilator, this decrease of the tidal volume is the result of a large 'internal compliance'.

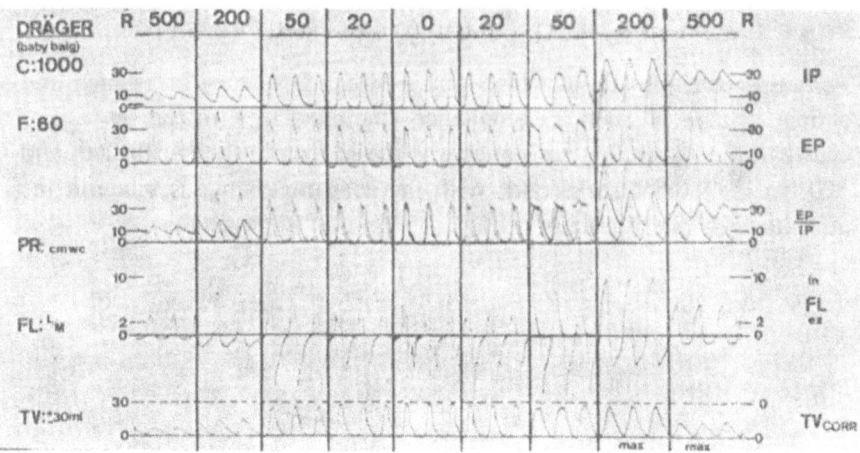

Dräger ventilator: The Dräger ventilator, even when provided with the small bellows for use with infants, shows the same picture as the Engström apparatus. Read from the middle column (O), leftwards, no change was made in the settings of the ventilator. Read toward the right, the record reflects an attempt to compensate for the loss of tidal volume by modification of the adjustment, which was not entirely successful. At the highest resistance (R 500) the ventilation pressure (EP) amounts to 40 cm H_2O, which is not an exceptional value. After the correction it reaches even 70 cm H_2O, at which the starting value of 30 ml is still not reached. Here too, the high internal compliance takes its effect.

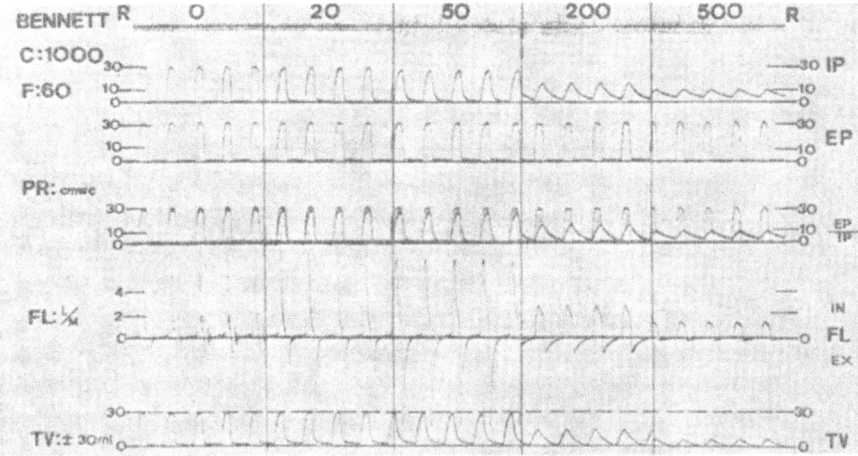

Bennet ventilator: This is a typical example of a pressure-cycled ventilator. The ventilation pressure (EP) is constant. At a load of R 50, the pressure in the lungs decreases slightly, and at R 200 and R 500 the tidal volume shows a distinct decrease to 40 and 20 per cent of the starting value, respectively.

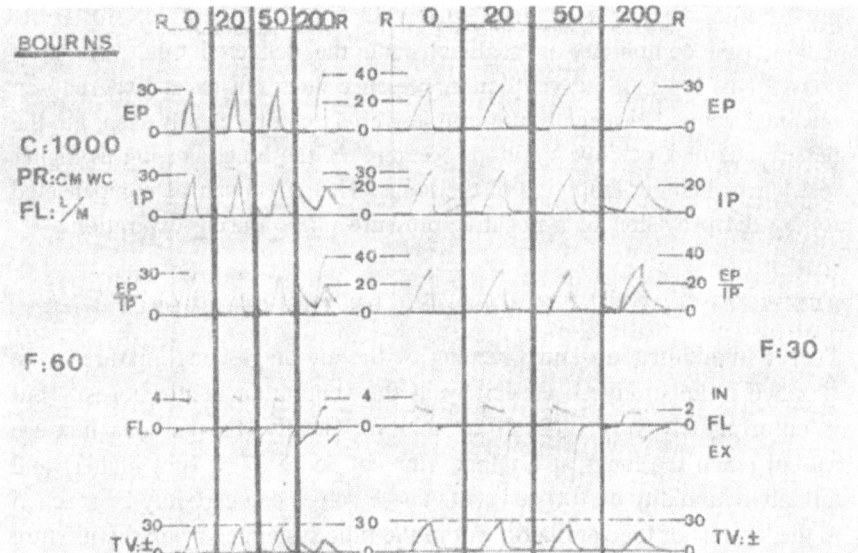

Bourns ventilator: The Bourns ventilator is specially constructed for use with infants. The R 500 resistance is not applied. As a result of the volume of the tube system and the humidifier, however, the internal compliance is so high that the tidal volume drops even at a load of R 50 and is reduced by half at R 200.

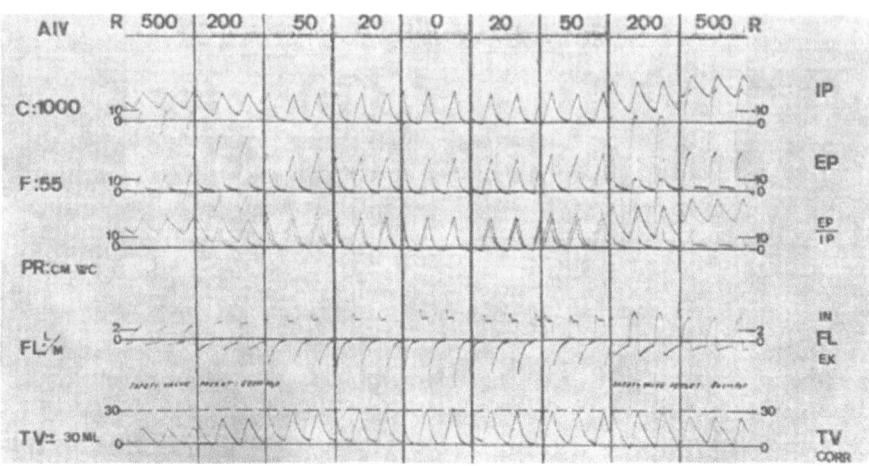

Amsterdam infant ventilator: This machine is designed for newborn and premature infants. Read from the middle column (0) leftwards, the adjustment was unchanged. The safety valve was set at a pressure of 50 cm H_2O. The tidal volume remains constant up to a load of R 50. Read to the right, the safety valve setting was at a higher value (80 cm) and the pre-set tidal volume was maintained with a resistance of R 200. Here, the internal compliance is negligible and the delivered tidal volume is constant as long as the ventilation pressure does not exceed the chosen maximal value. Here again, the trapping effect can be clearly seen, i.e. the persistance of a positive 'residual pressure' in the lung, as soon as higher resistances hamper emptying of the lungs. This effect can be compensated for by the provision of a negative-pressure phase during expiration.

HUMIDIFICATION AND WARNING OF THE AIR SUPPLY

Proper humidification and warming of the air or gaseous mixture to be supplied is imperative – especially in the ventilation of newborns – but is unfortunately very difficult to achieve. Ideally, the gaseous mixture should reach the lungs at a temperature of 35 to 37°C (not higher) and a relative humidity of 100 per cent. These values can certainly be reached at the 'egress' of the ventilator, but in the tube system carrying the mixture to the infant the gas cools off; the water vapour condenses and the mixture reaches the child with a relative humidity of 100 per cent but at a lower temperature. The only solution is to take a still higher input temperature, e.g. 50°C, but this makes it necessary to retrieve the excess water before it can reach the baby and, furthermore, to measure and record the temperature of the gas at the place at which it reaches the trachea. Condensation can be substantially reduced by having as little as possible of the tube system outside the incubator and as much as possible of it inside the incubator.

The best method to humidifiy the gaseous mixture is the addition of water vapour, which can give a better guarantee of sterility. Aerosolization, even when achieved ultrasonically, entails a risk of infection and there is considerable chance that unknown amounts of water are supplied to the child. Cases have been reported in which a 'water intoxication' resulted from this procedure.

Recently, a thorough study of the humidification capacity of various humidifiers suitable for use with a ventilator has been published (Hayes and Robertson, *Brit. J. Anaesth.* 1970, vol. 42, no. 2, 94). In this investigation the relative humidity was measured after the gas had been heated to 37°C. The results are, as could be expected, dependent on the gas flow. For the ventilation of infants this value seldom exceeds 6 litres/min, and for prematures even lies around 1 litre/min.

Taken from this study, the following are the values found for several well-known humidifiers suitable for use in combination with a ventilator. For the reasons already mentioned, the nebulizers are not included.

Humidifier	Gas flow (litres/min)	Relative humidity at 37°C (%) (dependent on use of low-flow cartridge and nebulizer)
Cape ventilator	10	60
Amst. infant vent.	2	72
Bennett Cascade	10	70—76
Air Shields PN 49	4	47
Puritan Heated Ned.	10	32

When humidification is applied, it is imperative to measure the temperature of the inhaled gaseous mixture at the place where it flows into the trachea and to provide for warning of the supply tubes to prevent condensation. If condensation does occur, the precipitation must be eliminated before it can reach the lungs.

ARTIFICIAL VENTILATION OF INFANTS

J. J. VAN ZANTEN

It seemed logical to apply mechanical ventilation not only to adults and children with respiratory difficulties but also to infants. For our first cases we ventilated with the Bird apparatus via an oral endotracheal or a tracheostomy tube, but it soon became evident that the method would have to be modified to make it suitable for these small patients.

There are still practitioners who give preference to the primary tracheostomy for the ventilation of infants. For this purpose and for the bronchial aspiration the use of a tracheostomy tube indeed gives an easier approach than an endotracheal tube. But decannulation sometimes gives difficulties: for instance the mechanism by which the glottis is opened during respiration does not function, or hypoplasia of the larynx has developed, or the tracheal wall weakened by the tracheostoma is pulled inward at inspiration and closes off the trachea, or a tracheal stenosis develops.

The oral endotracheal tube is, except for ventilation lasting only a few hours, unusable. It cannot be properly fixed and therefore moves in the mouth, thus involving the risk of occlusion due to bending, of dislocation, and of injury to the vocal cords.

From almost the beginning we have used a plastic nasotracheal tube without a cuff to ventilate infants, initially the Jackson-Rees tube, later the Rüsch tube. After a little practice, nasotracheal intubation can be performed rapidly and easily. Good external fixation is required to prevent the tube from coming to lie too deep or not deep enough. Because it runs through the nose, the motility of the tube is additionally limited. We do not change the tube routinely every few days; the adhesion of thick secretions in the tube can usually be prevented by adequate humidification of the inspired gas, the occasional application of mucolytic agents in the tube, and frequent performance of bronchial aspiration. Furthermore, since the plastic material does not irritate, the tube can in any case be left in place for fourteen days without damage to the vocal cords or larynx.

158

If ventilation is required for much longer than fourteen days, a tracheostomy is performed as well – although in prematures we sometimes leave the nasotracheal tube *in situ* for a month. We have seen only one case in which a severe fibrous stenosis developed, at the level of the cricoid, due to the presence of a nasotracheal tube; this was the first neonate whom we ventiliated, because the lungs were not aerated. At that time we were still using the Bird ventilator, and we only succeeded in expanding the lungs by using a tube of a size that was much too large for a child of his age. Because of the stenosis he could not be discharged, although he was otherwise completely healthy and was developing normally. Emergency intubation was repeatedly necessary, sometimes combined with cardiac massage, because of total occlusion of the trachea. At the age of 2½, just when plans had been completed for a surgical reconstruction of the trachea, his breathing and heart-beat stopped again, after which he remained comatose until his death at the age of 3 years.

The normal nasotracheal tube size for a newborn has an internal diameter of 2.5 mm. Bronchial aspiration via this tube is a far from simple procedure; even if the child itself is able to breathe, he is prevented from doing so because the moistened suction catheter, which has an external diameter of 1.66 mm., almost completely blocks the tube, and at the same time air is also sucked out of the lungs via the suction catheter (with a faulty technique, this suction can even lead to atelectastis of a lobe). Consequently, the bronchial toilet must be done quickly and adequately, with one eye on the ECG monitor to anticipate hypoxic bradycardia. By means of bronchial aspiration combined with good humidification of the inspired gas, vibration of the thorax, and regularly alternating the child's position from one side to the other, the air passages can be cleared and atelectasis abolished or prevented.

Since 1966 we have ventilated infants with the Amsterdam Infant Ventilator designed by Keuskamp, a volume-constant apparatus capable of reaching a high respiratory frequency. On a few occasions we have used this apparatus as a pressure-constant ventilator to obtain a pressure plateau and improved gas distribution, but under this condition a constant alveolar ventilation is not guaranteed.

A normal pCO_2 can usually be maintained easily. But to obtain an acceptable oxygen saturation of, for example, about 90 per cent (pO_2 60 mm Hg), the child must often be ventilated for a long period with 60 to 80 per cent O_2 in the inspired gas. The high oxygen concentration is present only in the air passages and the lungs, which can lead to local complications, of which I may mention a few:

1. Resorption atelectasis of hypoventilated alveolae, resulting in a further decrease in the oxygen saturation due to 'relative' right-left shunts.
2. Decreasing vibrissal movement and mucus flow in the trachea (observed by Laurenzi et al., 1968, in cats).
3. (Only in premature infants.) Bronchopulmonary dysplasia with peribronchial and later alveolar fibroblast proliferation, resulting in impeded ventilation and decreasing oxygen saturation. Radiographically, the picture can sometimes be recognized: initially, course granular infiltrates are present; later, small cyst-like radiolucencies are seen in the lungs.

In some cases a high inspiratory pressure ($+$ 45 cm H_2O) is required for a considerable length of time to maintain alveolar ventilation. This may lead to impedance of the venous return and possibly of the pulmonary bloodflow. Pneumothorax due to rupture in an emphysematous area, due to irregular ventilation, rarely occurs.

Work is in progress on a monitor for the Amsterdam Infant Ventilator, to signal respiratory failure and excessively high inspiratory pressures.

Proper humidification of the inspired gas, to replace the physiological moistening via the nasal mucosa and to prevent the drying out of sputum and bronchial secretions, can be achieved best with the heated humidifier belonging to the Amsterdam Infant Ventilator. The so-called artificial nose or humidity condenser gives very inadequate humidification: after one to three days the thick bronchial secretion is almost impossible to remove.

A neonate that has been ventilated for several days often remains apnoeic when the artifical ventilation is terminated: his blood-gas values are normal and he lies in a warm incubator, so that a respiratory stimulus is lacking. By the time that the rising pCO_2 and the decreasing pH level would start to provide this stimulus, severe hypoxia has already developed and the respiratory centre can no longer react to the adequate stimulus. In some cases the child's breathing can be started immediately after the termination of mechanical ventilation by the application of external stimulae. It is also possible to provide a respiratory stimulus in the form of a light metabolic or respiratory acidosis or by the administration of prethcamidum, before terminating mechanical ventilation. Provision must be made that with the very first breath the child takes in a considerable amount of oxygen. After the termination of ventilation the nasotracheal tube is usually left in place for another day under continuous observation.

After removal of the nasotracheal tube, oedema of the glottis may develop. In view of the narrowness of the air passages, even a very slight amount of glottal oedema will impede breathing. The occurrence of oedema of the glottis is routinely prevented by spraying the vocal cords with Otrivin® every three hours for one day. After prolonged intubation we also administer corticosteroids to control glottal oedema. In a few cases it has been necessary to continue this corticosteroid treatment for more than a month.

During and after ventilation, continuous ECG and heart-rate monitoring are imperative. Thorax radiograms and blood-gas analyses are made routinely. On the basis of the SaO_2 values obtained from gas analysis of blood samples from the heel and the hand, it is possible to determine whether a right-left shunt via a still-open ductus Botalli is present.

CLINICAL RESULTS

Since 1965, a total of 119 infants have been ventilated in the Intensive Care Unit of the Leiden University Hospital. Of these, 84 died. This high mortality is partially ascribable to the underlying condition, which proved retrospectively to be untreatable, e.g. cerebral haemorrhages in neonates and certain congenital heart diseases. Furthermore, the child's condition had often been poor for some time before admission for ventilation, due for instance to respiratory and circulatory failure, shock, hypoxia (sometimes with an SaO_2 of 30 per cent), acidosis (not infrequently with a pH of 6.9 or lower), and hypoglycaemia.

From the point of view of ventilation techniques, the differences between newborns and older infants are not very large, but there is an appreciable difference in the underlying disease. Most of the older ventilated infants had congenital heart defects. Most of those under seven days old had pulmonary anomalies or cerebral haemorrhages or both.

A total of 51 infants older than seven days were ventilated, of which 30 succumbed (60 per cent) (table 1). I shall not discuss these cases here, but confine myself to the infants with an age of less than seven days.

Table 1. Infants ventilated at ages over 7 days.

Underlying condition	Number succumbed	Number surviving
Cardiac diseases	21	19
Cerebral haemorrhage/meningitis	6	–
Other anomalies	3	2
Total	30	21

Ventilation was applied to 68 infants below seven days of age, of which 54 succumbed (80 per cent) (table 2).

Table 2. Infants ventilated at ages below 7 days.

Underlying condition	Number succumbed	Number surviving
Pulmonary diseases	4 (4)*	10 (6)
'Traumatic' cerebral haemorrhage	7 (1)	–
Pulmonary + 'traumatic' cer. haem.	12 (10)	1
Pulmonary + subependymal haemor. with ventricular haemor.	15 (14)	–
Cardiac diseases	8 (2)	–
'Neonatal shock'	–	1
Other anomalies	8 (5)	2 (1)
Total	54 (36)	14 (7)

* Values between parentheses pertain to prematures.

The four infants indicated as having died of pulmonary causes include the infant described above, which had made a good recovery but died at the age of three years due to a tracheal stenosis.

The smallest premature infant ventilated had a birth weight of 625 grams, and the smallest ventilated premature infant that survived weighed 940 grams at admission.

Table 2 does not include cases of infants with hydrops foetalis; these children had on the one hand a glottal oedema impeding or preventing respiration and on the other elevation of the diaphragm due to the hepatosplenomegaly, the ascites, and the blood transfusions given intra-uterinely. In these cases ventilation was generally required for only a few hours and was performed during the first substitution transfusion in the department of gynaecology.

It seems worth-while to discuss the pulmonary anomalies and cerebral haemorrhages in neonates in more detail.

PULMONARY ANOMALIES

The diagnosis hyaline membranes can only be made with certainty histologically. Clinically, only the probable diagnosis can be reached. Many of the studies done on hyaline membranes are unreliable because the diagnosis was based on post mortem evidence. Clinically, it is only possible to establish that radiologically the lungs are insufficiently aerated, that breathing requires great effort, that the oxygen saturation is reduced, and that acidosis is present, often more metabolic than respiratory. A more exact differentiation of this picture is possible and useful:

1. From birth the lungs are badly aerated, for instance because of aspiration of amniotic fluid, because the child has not cried hard enough (caesarian section, depression of respiration due to medicaments admistered to the mother), or inadequate pulmonary bloodflow. Particularly neonatal shock with inadequate pulmonary bloodflow, pulmonary vasoconstriction, and maintenance of the foetal circulation by a right-left shunt via the ductus Botalli, may sometimes play an important part in the failure of lung expansion.
2. Primary and adequate lung expansion with a decrease in the aeration of the lungs starting about six hours after birth. These are conceivably the 'true' cases of hyaline membrane.

CEREBRAL HAEMORRHAGE

An infant with a cerebral haemorrhage should not be ventilated: even if he can be kept alive, his cerebral anomalies will make it impossible for him to lead a human existence. Of the 54 deceased neonates in our material, 34 had had a cerebral haemorrhage, and it is perhaps permissible to say that it was right that these children died.

The clinical diagnosis cerebral haemorrhage is difficult to arrive at because:

- Grunting during expiration is also seen in pulmonary anomalies.
- Dullness, atonia, fluttering movements of the extremities and periodic apnoea can be caused by anoxia, acidosis, and hypoglycaemia.
- Attacks of apnoea also occur in premature infants with an 'unripe' respiratory centre.
- Very suspicious clinically, is the infant that initially shows normal respi-

ration and then suddenly becomes periodically apnoeic while the thorax radiogram, the blood-gas analyses, and the blood-sugar level remain normal.

– When possible, before the child has reached the point of requiring ventilation, the presence or absence of a cerebral haemorrhage should be demonstrated on the basis of material obtained by lumbar puncture.

In emergency situations, however, ventilation will often be started before a cerebral haemorrhage has been diagnosed. The well-ventilated infant with a cerebral haemorrhage often shows (virtually) no neurological anomalies. The first indication of an increasing cerebral haemorrhage is rather often in these cases an acute stubborn metabolic acidosis, probably based on inadequate circulation.

The cause of the 'traumatic' cerebral haemorrhage is clear, but the cause of subependymal haemorrhage is less distinct; it is usually considered to be a result of anoxia, in part because of its frequent occurrence in combination with pulmonary anomalies. On the other hand, there are many cases of traumatic cerebral haemorrhage combined with pulmonary anomalies, and consequently the common cause may well lie in the prematurity. We certainly have no idea how many children there are with a strictly local subependymal haemorrhage. Two of our infants, who died from other causes, proved to have such local subependymal haemorrhages.

If a subependymal haemorrhage breaks through into the ventricles, which usually occurs within one to five days, the results are often fatal within a matter of hours, despite ventilation; but two of our cases showed a longer survival time (1½ and 4 months).

Assuming tentatively that the subependymal haemorrhage is indeed caused by anoxia, it must be concluded that in this case too, prompt oxygenation is imperative.

CONCLUSIONS

Ventilation certainly deserves a place in perinatal care. All cases with respiratory disorders that endanger life or can lead to secondary brain damage should be considered for ventilation if they do not respond properly to conservative treatment.

The possibility of a cerebral haemorrhage must be excluded if possible, since it seems wrong to keep an individual with such a hopeless prognosis alive artificially.

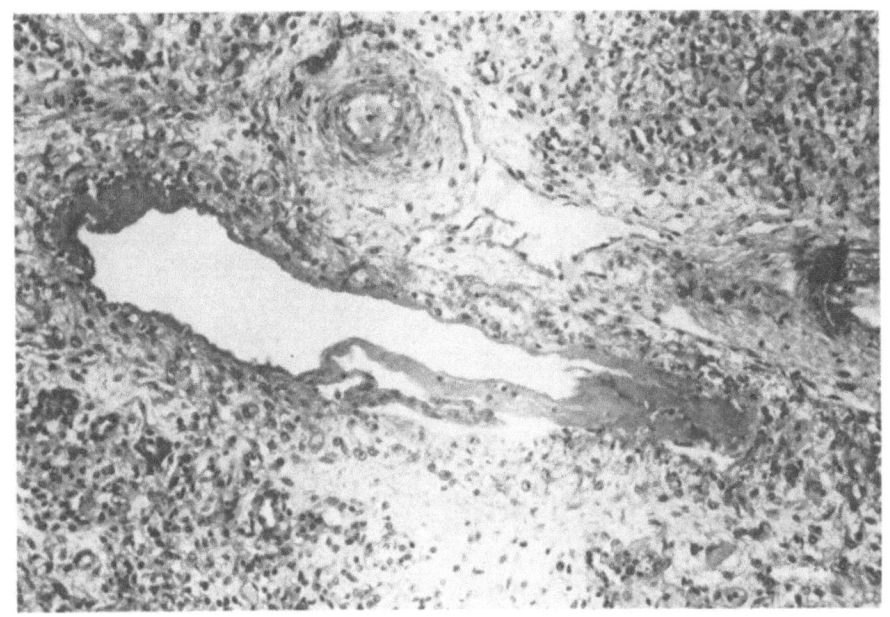

Fig. 1

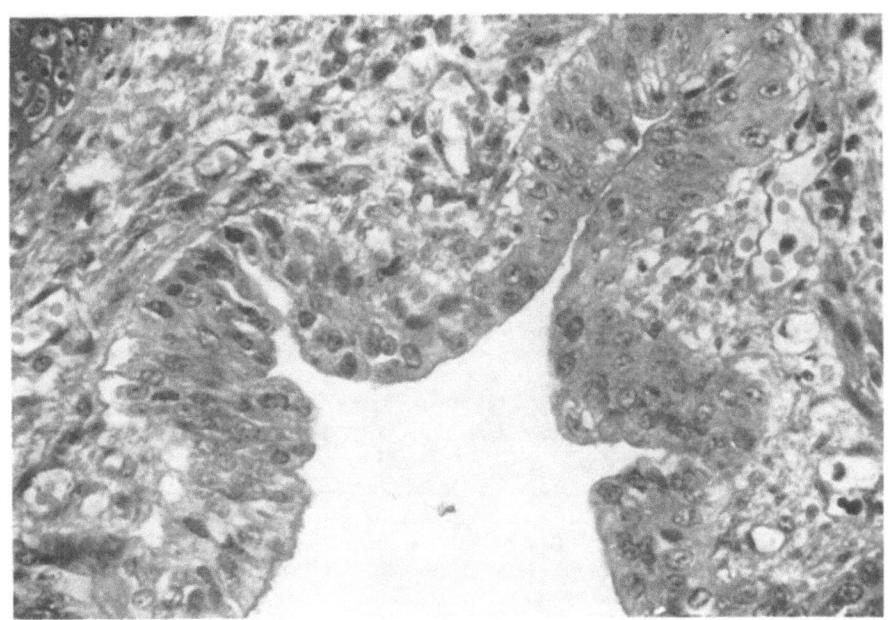

Fig. 2

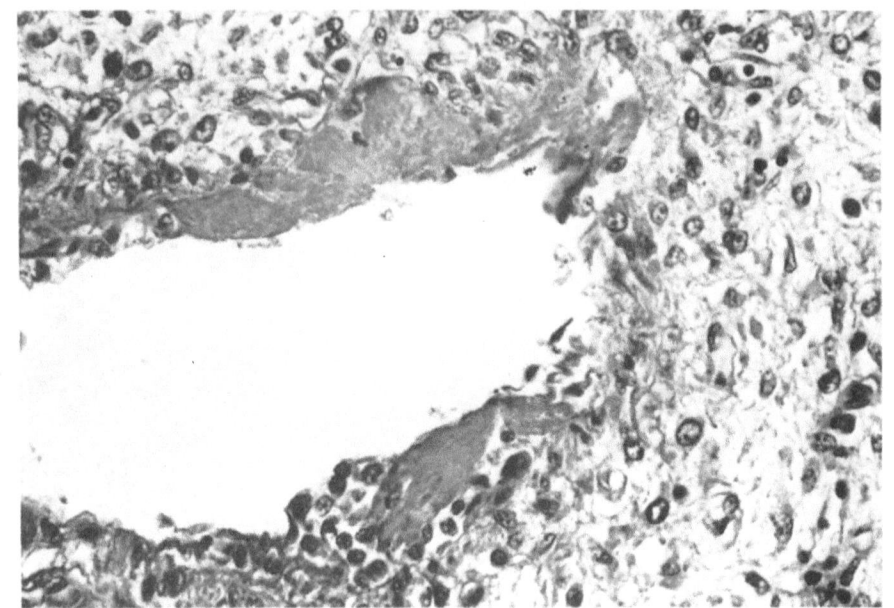

Fig. 3

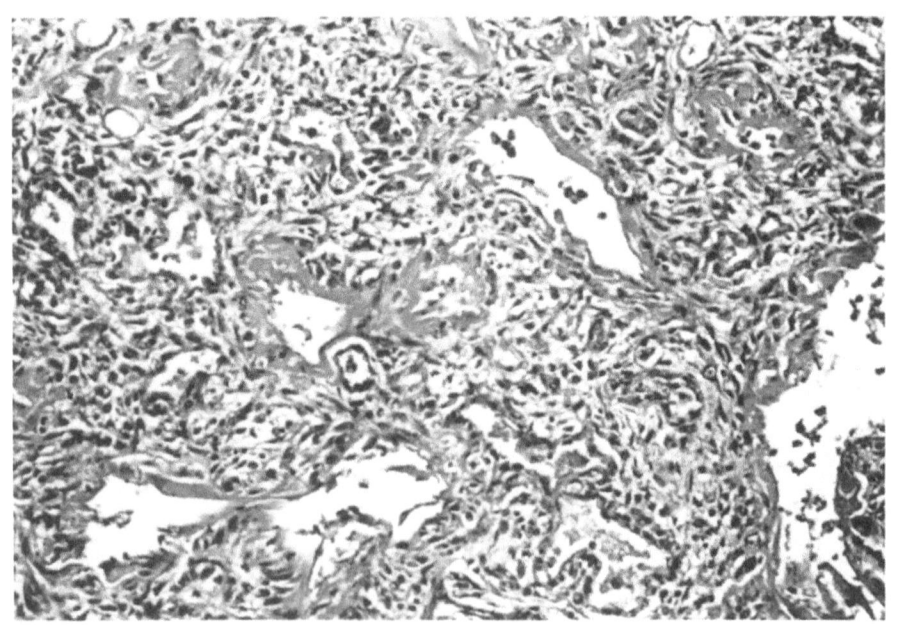

Fig. 4

PATHOLOGICAL FINDINGS IN VENTILATED NEWBORNS

J. L. J. GAILLARD

Autopsy was performed in 37 cases of children who had died under ventilation with oxygen-rich (60 to 80 per cent) gaseous mixtures because of respiratory disorders. The duration of the ventilation ranged from a few hours to 40 days. Twenty-seven of these children died in the neonatal period (first week), the other 10 at ages ranging from 9 days to 5 months. The relevant data of these cases is given in tables 1 and 2.

The pulmonary anomalies in children after oxygen-rich ventilation reported in the literature are known under the term 'bronchiolar dysplasia', which refers to the disturbance of the normal structure (dysplasia) of the bronchial epithelium; this is, however, only one of the morphological aspects of the picture. A reconstruction of the anomalies found in different patients makes the following pathogenesis probable:

1. epithelial destruction in small bronchial rami and bronchioli with deposition of fibrin on the bronchial wall (fig. 1);
2. excessive peribronchial edema (fig. 1);
3. regeneration of epithelium accompanied by dysplasia (fig. 2); and
4. proliferation of mesenchymal cells resembling fibroblasts and possible proliferation of capillaries (fig. 3 and 4).

This picture develops first peribronchially and peribronchiolarly, but after a few days of ventilation it also shows a diffuse perialveolar distribution in the lungs.

The presence of all or a part of this pathological picture seems to be correlated with the degree of prematurity of the infant (tables 1 and 2). When the picture occurs in infants born à term, the histological development of the kidneys proves to be premature. Conversely, when the picture is absent in pre-term born neonatally deceased children, the histological development of the kidneys is found to correspond with à term. These cases are indicated in tables 1 and 2 by an exclamation point in the

165

Table 1. Neonatal deaths under ventilation 1968–1969.

Age [1]	Duration of venti- lation [2]	Develop- ment [3]	Dysma- turity	Pul- monary anomalies	Pathology
4	a few hours	I	–	– !	intra-uter. pneumonia
1½	½	P	+	– !	mec. aspiration
1	¾	P	–	+	HMS [4]
1	1	P	–	+	HMS/Rhes.
2	1	P	–	+	HMS
2	1	P	–	+	HMS
1½	1	P	–	+	HMS
4	1½	P	–	+	HMS
5	1½	P	–	+	HMS
2	2	P	–	+	HMS
3	3	I	–	+	HMS
4	3	P	–	+	HMS
7	4	P	–	+	HMS ?
5	4¾	P	–	+	HMS
5	5	P	–	+	HMS
6	6	P	–	+	HMS
1	1	P	–	– !	still born mec. aspiration intra-uter. pneumonia
3	1½	P	+ histol. develop- ment mature (kidney)	– !	navel sepsis + pneumonia
5 hour	1 hour	M	–	–	birth trauma
1	a few hours	M	–	–	intra-uter. pneumonia
5	a few hours	M	–	–	heart defect
7	4 hour	M	–	–	ileumatresia
7	7 hour	M	–	–	heart defect
5	1	M	–	–	heart defect
7	6	M	–	–	mec. aspiration birth trauma
4	4	M	+ histol. develop- ment premature (kidney)	+ !	mec. aspiration

Table 1 (continued)

Age [1]	Duration of venti-lation [2]	Develop-ment [3]	Dysma-turity	Pul-monary anomalies	Pathology
7	6	M	+ histol. develop-ment premature (kidney)	+ !	hernia diaphr. + pneumonia

[1] Age in days, unless otherwise indicated.
[2] Duration in days, unless otherwise indicated.
[3] I = immature
  P = premature
  M = mature
[4] Hyaline membrane syndrome

Table 2. Infant deaths under ventilation 1968–1969.

Age [1]	Duration of venti-lation [2]	Develop-ment [3]	Dysma-turity	Pul-monary anomalies	Pathology
150	6	P	–	+	heart defect
14	12	P	–	+	hernia diaphr. pneumonia
41	40	I	–	+	subep. bleeding
9	8	P	+ hist. develop-ment premature (kidney)	+	clin. toxicosis caesarean section
35	2½	P	+ hist. develop-ment mature (kidney)	– !	heart defect
13	a few hours	M	–	–	heart defect
21	a few hours	M	–	–	heart defect
12	5	M	–	–	heart defect
12	7	M	–	–	heart defect
9	8	M	–	–	mec. aspiration

[1] Age in days, unless otherwise indicated
[2] Duration in days, unless otherwise indicated
[3] I = immature   P = premature   M = mature

pulmonary-anomaly column. The first two patients mentioned in table 1 were ventilated for only a very short time, and consequently no morphologically visible pulmonary anomalies are to be expected.

Ventilation experiments with healthy mice born pre-term and *à term* have shown that similar pulmonary anomalies can be induced, but only when the gaseous mixture contains 80 to 100 per cent oxygen (Rosan). Furthermore, there is a distinct positive correlation with the prematurity of these animals (pre-term group). The presence of a particular lung disease is not required for the development of the picture.

Although the number of cases in our material is not large, a few conclusions can be cautiously drawn:

1. A high percentage of oxygen seems to be a causal condition for the development of the picture of so-called bronchiolar dysplasia.
2. The genesis of the anomalies is probably not causally correlated with the nature of the underlying disease process in the lungs, such as the hyaline membrane syndrome, pneumonia, or aspiration of amniotic fluid with or without meconium.
3. In all likelihood, the functional prematurity of an infant at the time of ventilation is an important condition for the development of the picture seen in the lungs.

The results of our investigation are supported by the previously reported experimental observations in mice. It therefore seems probable that the high local oxygen concentration in the lungs, in combination with the prematurity of the child, can lead to the picture of so-called bronchiolar dysplasia.

REFERENCE

Rosan R., Paediatric Pathology Society, meeting New Castle, 1969.

SUMMING-UP

H. H. VAN GELDEREN

I feel honoured by the invitation to provide a summarizing comment on this course, especially because I am not a neonatologist. As Dr. Ruys has said in introducing me, this may be an advantage because the contents of this course can be reviewed from some distance.

In my opinion the course on an important subject in medicine has been constructed as it should be. You have been able to listen to a number of various representants of different specialities. Also the listeners themselves consist of members of various disciplines. The ultimate aim of all the work which has been discussed here is clear: in which way can we reach a maximal reduction of perinatal mortality and morbidity in the light of present knowledge and possibilities. Morbidity is not only restricted to the perinatal period but includes all the possible later sequelae of damage originating from the period around birth. I added the words: in the light of present knowledge and possibilities, because these are limiting factors.

Distribution of knowledge is the 'raison d'être' of all Boerhaave-courses. Though every lecture that you have heard was a separate small chapter of perinatal physiology or pathology, capita selecta et nova from a much wider area of research and clinical science, I think the construction of the course has become clear to you. Physiologists and biochemists have presented some back-ground knowledge and they were followed by clinicans with presentation of more or less profound clinical research. Treatment of respiratory disease, hypoxia-acidosis and hypoglycaemia has been discussed also with regard to the technical implications. At the end the pathologists have told us what can be learnt from those cases in whom the clinician has lost the struggle.

A course like this can only deal with a restricted number of problems but in my opinion the main line has been maintained throughout. I also think

169

that we all have been served well, though we belong to so many different disciplines. Usually, at least in this hospital, this type of courses are called integrated courses. In my opinion this is not true. The course itself is not integrated, but we hope that you will be able as listeners to integrate the subjects which have been discussed.

The first lecture by the well-known physiologist Dawes contained a highly interesting explanation about the physiology of the placenta. This lecture was very useful also to the clinician and in general to everybody who has the care of newborn children and unborn children. I especially think of his relativating the significance of the placenta as an organ for gas exchange, and of the stress he has put on the metabolism of the placenta itself with its large oxygen consumption and CO_2 production. His findings about the placenta-flow, the many factors which influence this flow, even to such an extent that the foetus may suffer, and the important fact that flow through the uterine artery should not be considered equal to the placenta-flow, all these are important facts. The data from experimental investigations are of great interest, not only for increasing our knowledge, but especially for those who are planning investigations of placental function themselves, because it remains a very difficult task to study the function of the placenta. They may prevent hasty conclusions and simple model-thinking.

At the end of his lecture Dr. Dawes has indicated the great importance of aortic receptors whose efferent tracks are contained in the vagus nerve.

The lecture of Dr. Eskes also belongs to a certain extent to clinical physiology. His data about the pressure relationship between parts of the uterus and its contents lead a.o. to the important conclusion about the homogeneous pressure distribution in the whole uterus. His comparisons with lunar capsules and diving reactions of the seal were rather humorous though – as appeared from the discussion – they have their restrictions. The presentation of computer analyses of the registration of heartfrequency of the unborn child can give us an idea of the improvement of information deducted from registration of heart action during birth.

The only biochemist among the speakers, Dr. Shelley, also aimed to increase or revive our knowledge of more fundamental processes. It is always good to be reminded again of the fact that glucose is virtually the only source of energy for the foetus. This is one of the reasons why hypoxia is so dangerous because it may lead easily to lactic acidosis which in itself may be fatal. Her plea for administration of glucose and alcali during the birth-process in case of hypoxia is worth a trial (it has been tried already in some centres), though only if careful chemical control is possible. Dr. Shelley stressed the significance of the usually large stores of glycogen. We should not only think of liver glycogen in this respect but also of the glycogen present in heart and muscle as a source of glucose in the first hours after birth. The importance of glycogen stores outside the liver has been known to paediatricians from the fact that children with glycogen storage disease usually do not have difficulties shortly after birth.

Dr. Popescu, an anaesthetist, discussed distribution and transport of barbiturates, local anaesthetics, and some other drugs. His lecture also could be grouped under those lectures which aimed at increasing our knowledge of more basal processes. His beautiful way of explaining made it very easy for us to follow him, though for many of us it must have been many years ago when we listened to lectures about pharmacodynamics. The great significance of the way of administration of drugs, the variations in distribution among the tissues, the influence of circulation, the different ways these drugs pass the placenta as well as the great importance of the factor time when checking concentrations, all this demonstrates clearly how little we know and especially how much we do not take into account when we treat the mother with anaesthetics and other drugs. This again stresses the risk to the unborn child which may be associated with all forms of medical treatment of the mother. In any case it is clear that much investigation in this area is necessary and that simplification in this type of work may be dangerous.

With the lecture of Dr. Gevers about the work of his group of obstetricians we reached the clinic. He explained to us how his data about foetal heart frequency, pH, HCO_3^- and glucose levels of foetal blood during and after birth, the condition of the child and the kind of parturition relate with each other. These data confirm that examination of foetal blood during and after birth is very important both for guiding the parturition as for the prediction of the condition of the child in the first hours after birth. To his opinion monitoring the heart frequency does not give much additional information, though it may be of some use in indicating the need to investigate the blood of the child. From the discussions you will have learned that the foetal heart-monitoring-fans, as we could call them, did not accept this opinion meekly. As far as I could conclude from the discussions it still is not proved that foetal heart-monitoring is of great use in predicting the condition of the child at birth. But it is possible that computeranalysis and further experiences may change this. I do think that there is a need for more data of the type Dr. Gevers group have been collecting. Then statistical analysis can be performed which will not only give more exact information but also may result in a more practical guide for the physician who cannot dispose of all the facilities which are available to workers in an university hospital. It is quite possible that a good analysis of all results will show that with less determinations useful information can still be obtained.

The lecture of Dr. Spierdijk has fixed our attention upon the possible influence which variations of the acid-base equilibrium in the mother may have upon the foetus. Hyperventilation of the mother, as Dawes had already mentioned earlier, may led to hypoxia and acidosis of the child. Whether this is a direct chemical relationship, as Spierdijk suggests, is open to question. In any case the anaesthetist has an important task in the prevention of both hypoxia and hyperventilation in the mother. Perhaps in this respect I may say a word for the kidney. Prof. Spierdijk has said that it may last many hours before compensation of acidosis or alkalosis by the kidney starts. To my opinion the kidney is not so lazy, and will act much earlier upon changes of acidbase equilibrium. This is not to suggest that determination of urinary pH is an important or useful method in treatment of disturbances of acid-base equilibrium in the mother, because it is not.

Dr. Kubli discussed the influence of oxytocin on the child, and gave a lot of important information. I should like especially to remind you of his conclusion that it is not always a safe drug to give as an intravenous infusion and may lead to hypoxia of the foetus. This has also been stressed in the discussion after his lecture. The intravenous route can be used safely only in case one can registrate continuously uterine contractions, which of course cannot be done outside a few centres. However it is up to the obstetrician to decide in which way the information presented by Dr. Kubli will influence the further use of oxytocin-infusions.

The paper of Dr. Ruys appeared to me to be a clear, succinct and practical presentation of treatment of anoxic newborns. It reads like a manual for the doctor in charge of a neonatal unit. From the neonatal mortality figures in his unit it is clear, that the manual will be a good one. There remain of course a number of suggestions about which the discussion has not yet been closed. I could mention e.g. the risk of strongly hyperosmolar infusions, the risk of hypocalcaemia, the interpretation of data deducted from pH measurements, the question whether capillary blood always represents the actual acid-base equilibrium and to what extent his method of treatment will prevent the respiratory distress syndrome. The last question seems pertinent, because it seems that the frequency of hyaline membrane disease in his unit is remarkably low. However, there is no doubt that his guide for treatment of the newborn is completely up-to-date and is strongly recommended.

Another paediatrician, Dr. de Leeuw, discussed the well-known problem of neonatal hypoglycaemia. It was interesting to note that we still do not quite know what are the causes of this hypoglycaemia; we are also not yet sure why so often this hypoglycaemia does not react sufficiently on glucose administration. A few years ago in our country a symposium was held about this subject and the many questions posed at that time still cannot be answered. Dr. de Leeuw could not dwell upon the aetiology as time was restricted. There is a need for much more information about the role of insulin, growth hormone and adreno-cortical steroïds in the regulation of neonatal glucose blood levels. We may expect that in the next years more will become known about these problems. Dr. de Leeuw has stressed predisposing factors and in this respect his remark during discussion that, whatever the indications, glucose administration is safe, should be noted. It is clear that in high-risk children, predisposed to hypoglycaemia (especially small-for-date children) administration of glucose should be performed freely, even if one is not able to check blood glucose continuously or very frequently. Also feeding should not be unnecessarily be postponed. It is likely that a lot of serious problems can be prevented by this practical method.

The last day was mainly devoted to problems around artificial ventilation. Prof. Keuskamp who himself has done important work on construction of ventilators (one of which carries his name) gave a highly interesting paper about the methods of testing these instruments. He also gave an illuminating description of the special requirements attached to a ventilator for very young infants. Though clinicians usually do not have a good knowledge of the internal structure of the instruments they use, it is clear that it is very difficult to employ an infant ventilator without a good knowledge of requirements and construction of such an instrument.

Dr. van Zanten read a paper about the methods of artificial ventilation and the problems which are encountered in the special intensive-care department of this hospital. I think it should be clear to everybody that this form of advanced treatment should be confined to the few centers in the country which both can build up sufficient experience and have available sufficient trained personnel.

At the moment the results are still meagre in terms of survival rates, while indications for treatment are still uncertain. Very little information exists about late results; we still do not know what happens to the patients who survive the period of artificial ventilation. There is an urgent need here for good follow-up studies.

Dr. van Zanten has stressed the fact that the results can be improved, if we could refuse patients who most likely will not profit by this form of treatment and if we could confine ourselves to those who have a better prognosis.

This of course is quite true but it is not so simple. Especially we feel it is still difficult to recognize the patient whose respiratory distress either is caused by or is associated with intracranial haemorrhage. Hyaline membrane disease, once the clinical picture is well developped, can probably not be helped by artificial ventilation; but again it is not so easy to know when this stage has been reached and it is necessary to diagnose these patients earlier. It is therefore necessary for every center to analyse continuously patient material and the results. Also it will be important to transport highrisk children, that are those children of whom one can foresee that they probably will have to be ventilated, immediately to an intensive care unit. In this way one need not run the risk that the children will be sent too late and too hastily in a bad condition to the centre. Only those intensive care units, where artificial ventilation and other intensive care methods for treating newborns and prematures are possible, should accept these children.

Many question the ethics of artificial ventilation of newborns, because they fear most of the children who survive will be severely brain damaged. I doubt whether this problem is as large as some make us believe. Anyway, every form of advanced treatment which may result in survival of severely damaged children will also prevent severe damage in other children. Though it is nearly impossible to weigh these advantages and disadvantages, there is no reason to suppose that advanced treatment of newborns will increase the total number of children with severe brain damage.

Dr. Gaillard's lecture was the last one of this course. He has demonstrated to you pathological abnormalities of the premature lung, which are almost certainly the consequence of artificial ventilation and high concentrations of oxygen. During the discussion this problem of lung damage caused by treatment was further elucidated by Dr. Rosen, who has done experimental animal work on this problem. It is still not known, but it should be studied in the next years, whether this severe lung pathology also occurs in the children surviving treatment, whether they are clinicaly important and whether they will give rise to lungfibrosis. This again stresses the need of a very careful follow-up of patients who survive the advanced treatment during the first days of life. It is also necessary to check whether lower concentrations of oxygen during ventilation will prevent this pathology.

We have made acquaintance with both theoretical and practical new ideas and work. The question may be posed whether this all will bring us nearer to the goal, viz. a further reduction of mortality and morbidity of newborns. Maybe we should for the moment remain modest, because so much is still unknown. We still have to prove to what extent all these advancements of knowledge and treatment will be really effective in this respect. As said before we need very accurate analyses of mortality and morbidity as well as follow-up studies. Of course we are full of hope and it is very likely that the methods indicated and recommended by the speakers of this course will lead to the goal. However it remains important to prove this and to recognize possible wrong roads of advancement. Because there may be dangers attached to new methods of diagnosis and treatment.

In the first place, so called iatrogenic damage, the damage caused by investigation or treatment itself. This point has been stressed several times, especially during the last day.

In the second place, too much enthousiasm for instruments, tracings, laboratory results etc. without concurrent clinical evaluation. We know too well those patients, who according to the biochemical results from the laboratory are doing very fine but who are nevertheless dying. As Prof. Sikkel and others have said during this course, new methods and new instruments, for the moment at least, cannot replace good doctors and trained nurses.

The third danger is inexperience. It may be dangerous to start new methods of diagnosis and treatment or to follow recommendations of others, if one knows or should know that one will have neither the time nor the number of patients necessary to get experience and to keep up with the rapid evolution of medicine. Because of this the question which specialist: anaesthetist, obstetrician, pediatrician or whoever it may be, should treat the newborn and should perform resuscitation is not relevant. This only depends on whether the doctor appointed to it can do it well, has experience and is within reach at any time of the day and night. The question of diploma should not be the bone of contention as it still is in not so few hospitals.

And then, we should not forget the question of expertness. Everybody can buy apparatus and instruments if he takes the trouble. One should however also be able to interpret expertly the results given by the instruments and especially those of biochemical registration. One should also know exactly the reliability of these results.

In nearly all Boerhaave courses we meet the question of doctors in practice: what and how much can I do or should I do with the restricted possibilities to my disposal? I think you should not expect the right answer of university workers, they are probably the last ones who can give you a satisfactory answer. Doctors in the field should determine themselves in what way they should adapt a new and often difficult and expensive technic and should bear in mind the above mentioned dangers. They should refrain from adopting methods which have not as yet proved their efficacy. Personally I think these doctors in the field could get the best answer by following a stage in a university or comparable hospital. This form of post-graduate practical teaching in my view is very fertile and may be made possible by bilateral exchange transactions. After all if one cannot apply the most modern methods, this is not always a disadvantage. There may be a good chance that the method will be abandoned after some time. Sometimes it is not bad to be a few years behind, and to wait for long-term results, to sit on the fence so to speak.

May I finish by expressing the hope that this summing up will have strengthened the favourable judgement you no doubt have made about the quality of this Boerhaave course as well as about its benefits for the participants.

PANEL DISCUSSION

MODERATOR J. H. RUYS

Professor Keuskamp took the floor to answer questions addressed to him.

Koppe: What frequency do you advise for the Amsterdam Infant Ventilator? Are you of the opinion that low frequency with high pressure gives a better pO_2 than high frequency with low pressure?

Keuskamp: That depends entirely on the circumstances involved. In principle, a low respiration frequency is always better, because dead space has less influence, although with this apparatus the dead space is virtually absent. But if you have a low frequency, you also have a longer inspiration phase. And that is important because it gives a better and equal distribution of the inspired volume over a lung, with an uneven compliance in the lung itself. The only limitation of the low respiration frequency is that a certain minute volume cannot be escaped. If at this low respiration frequency a high tidal volume must be given at an abnormally high pressure, one is forced to raise the frequency. But this choice of frequency can never be predicted; it must actually be done with one's hand on the knob and one's eye on the child. This is the only possible solution.

Koppe: Is the Amsterdam Ventilator also suitable for use by the obstetrician in the delivery room for the ventilation of asphyctic newborns?

Keuskamp: Yes, in principle, since in place of an endotracheal tube an ordinary mask can be applied. But for this purpose you do not really need the whole apparatus. You can equally well use a normal mask and a so-called Ayre's system with an ordinary oxygen flow-meter, because a gas supply is needed in any case for the apparatus.

Question: An even distribution requires a minimal duration of the inspiration. I should be interested to hear your opinion as well as the experimental evidence if such exists.

Keuskamp: You must see the problem this way: if the inspiration lasts 0.2 second, a certain volume must enter in that 0.2 second. And this requires a high peak pressure, since without it that volume cannot be gotten into the lung. And this peak pressure distributes itself over the trachea and the bronchi. What you do with the very short inspiration time is ventilate not be alveoli but the bronchial tree, which in this short time expands too much.

Question: What is the limit of the very small respiratory volumes that you give? Is there a chance, in view of the fact that the lowest adjustment of the pump is 5 ml, that the administered tidal volume will be smaller than the dead space? Do you determine the dead space during ventilation and, if so, how?

Keuskamp: What is concerned is not the dead space of the newborn infant itself; the determining factor is the content of the endotracheal tube, which is about 1 to 1.5 ml. The dead space of the Amsterdam Ventilator is also about 1 ml, which gives in total a dead space as far as into the carina of about 2 ml. This must always be taken into account. The respiration volume you administer can be made as small as you wish, since it is dependent on the gas flow you use. This apparatus is also used in the pharmacological laboratory for the ventilation of mice and rats, which means that it can also be used to ventilate a premature infant.

Question: The inspiration flow-curve of the Amsterdam Ventilator does not have an S-shape. Is this not a disadvantage, and if so can the A.I.V. be modified to give an S-shaped inspiratory flow-curve?

Keuskamp: The Amsterdam Infant Ventilator is a constant flow generator, that is to say there is a horizontal plateau, as you could see from the drawings. What you would like to have is a plateau in the pressure curve. In other words, when the pressure rises plateau formation is obtained before the expiration. This can be favourable for a better distribution of the gasses in the lung at a given pressure. It can be obtained with this apparatus by allowing the pressure limiting valve to leak at a given pressure. But then you no longer know the tidal volume; you will have to guess at it, but that is not a serious drawback. The main thing is how the infant looks.

Question: What effect does leakage along the ventilation tube have on the constancy of the tidal volume?

Keuskamp: We speak of constant tidal volumes, but these are actually unattainable, because there is always leakage between the tube and the trachea. These small tubes are not cuffed, and this is a factor which must always be taken into account. It is quite possible that when you adjust the apparatus for a tidal volume of 20 ml, and certainly when there is a rather high inspiration pressure in the lung, that half of the expected 20 ml will leak back along the tube and escape. This forms one more argument that you can only ventilate under constant checking of the gas values and the infant's appearance. You must always expect leakage and always take it into account. With these extremely small tidal volumes and especially with the trend favouring the use of the smallest possible tubes having the least possible traumatic effect, leakages will of course always occur.

Van der Harten: Do you know anything about the type of expansion of the lung during ventilation in cases of the hyaline membrane disease? Is this of the centro-acinous type seen at autopsy?

Keuskamp: This is difficult to say, because for the newborn infants we have treated successfully there has been no autopsy and the pictures seen at autopsy are highly divergent, not only because the duration of the ventilation varies but also and mainly with respect to the moment at which ventilation was begun. These factors to a great extent determine the autopsy picture if the infant dies.

Dr. van Zanten answered questions addressed to him.

Hamming: What gas mixture is given preferentially for artificial ventilation of prematures: oxygen, nitrox, what percentage oxygen?

Van Zanten: Pure oxygen (100 percent) is given only in emergency situations for a very short time; in all other cases mixtures of oxygen and air, which is the simplest combination. It could also be called a mixture of oxygen and nitrogen. For these mixtures of oxygen and air we often require an oxygen percentage lying between 60 percent, with which we usually begin, and 80 percent if the situation deteriorates. The main point is not the percentage used for ventilation but rather the effect reached with it in the blood, for which certain criteria have been formulated: some consider a pO_2 of 50 mm Hg acceptable, others a pO_2 between 60 and 80. We prefer to reach an oxygen saturation value approaching 90 percent, which means a pO_2 of 60 mm Hg if the pH is normal. The problem concerns a clinical approach to the blood gas values more than the mixture supplied.

Van Aken: For bronchial aspiration in the ventilated infant do you make use of physiological saline or medicaments?

Van Zanten: We use Alévaire R, although that could equally well be physiological saline or bicarbonate. But we use (on the basis of experience) Alévaire R, added drop-wise in the tube, to dissolve drying secretions and to prevent them from sticking to the tube.

Van Aken: Is it possible to calculate the quantity of fluid administered to a ventilated infant via the humidifier?

Van Zanten: Yes, but in practice there are difficulties. You can in the first place measure the decrease in the water content of the humidifier over a certain period, and you must then also measure how much condensation water has remained in the tubes and in the ventilator. You must keep in mind that even if you do not supply any additional fluid to the infant in this way but simply replace the physiological moistening via the nasal mucosa by an artifical humidification, you nevertheless affect the water balance to a limited extent. Because normally, the infant inhales dry air, humidifies this air himself, and exhales air having a relative humidity of 100 percent at body temperature. Each breath drawn by an infant or adult therefore means a loss of water. This means that as soon as you introduce an external replacement for the physiological humidification by the nose, you are already supplying water.

Koppe: Is fluid introduced into the tube drop-wise additionally during ventilation? Or is this unnecessary when use is made of the heated humidifier plus the artificial nose?

Van Zanten: The first part of the question has already been answered. As to the second part, I did not think the idea was to use both. It is one or the other. The artifical nose is a kind of water isolator, the moisture being caught and condensed on gauze of a given pore size, so that at the next breath it is carried back to the infant. There is no point in inserting a water isolator between a humidifier and the infant, because the artificial nose forms a fluid barrier between the two.

De Bruijne: Are the speakers of the opinion that the heated humidifier gives adequate humidification?

Van Zanten: I cannot give an answer in concrete figures. I can only offer a clinical evaluation and say that we have obtained the impression that we can adequately prevent the drying up of secretions and that we certainly do not allow the lung to dry out. It is possible to state that an excess of fluid is supplied by the heated humidifier. But over the length of the tubes water of course condenses as the tubing cools, and one of the contrivances is to lay a large part of the Keuskamp tube in the incubator so that it remains more nearly at the right temperature. But even then, when the inspiration air has reached the infant its temperature will be somewhat lower than the body temperature in a number of cases, and under such conditions the humidification is no longer 100 percent.

De Steenhuijsen Piters: Have you had any experience with the Portex tubes, which in my opinion are made of a more pliant material than the Rüsch tubes and have a wider internal diameter?

Van Zanten: As far as the material is concerned, the Portex tubes are comparable to the Jackson-Reese tubes. You are correct with respect to the lumen and the plasticity. But the disadvantage is that just because of the plasticity there is also a chance that the tube will be pinched off at the approximately right angle it must pass between the floor of the nose and the trachea, and this is actually the only comment. It is not a fundamental objection. We find the Rüsch tubes somewhat better to work with, but if it were argued that the Portex or the Jackson-Reese is better, we could not object on demonstrable grounds.

De Steenhuijsen Piters: For the expansion of atelectatic areas do you use a prolonged (about 30 seconds) higher pressure repeated several times?

Van Zanten: Yes.

Question: Is humidification not accompanied by considerable condensation in the tube system?

Van Zanten: Yes; the tubes must be repeatedly evacuated to remove excess condensation fluid. This is a disadvantage, but it is more than outweighed by the advantage of the at least clinically good humidification.

Question: Have you had any experience with ultrasonic humidification in the respiratory circuit?

Van Zanten: Yes, in adults. Its disadvantage in infant ventilation is that in the small tubes used, turbulence of the gas flow leads to appreciably more condensation than normally occurs in an adult circuit and, furthermore, there is the disadvantage that an ultrasonic humidifier usually adds another lumen to the tube system, and as soon as the lumen of the apparatus and tube system becomes large in relation to the tidal volume it becomes more difficult to maintain a constant alveolar ventilation, certainly at high pressures, because part of the tidal volume is already compressed in the tube system and the lumen system of the apparatus.

Question: How do you collect arterial blood samples for the determination of pCO_2 and oxygen saturation?

Van Zanten: I do not collect them, or at least seldom; on rare occasions an arterial puncture is performed. But I need hardly say that for technical reasons this is not a simple matter, and we usually make use of arterialized blood from the heel or the hand or from combined punctures performed to exclude or demonstrate a ductus Botalli shunt from right to left.

De Leeuw: What do you take as indication for the ventilation of prematures?

Van Zanten: These indications must be arrived at gradually. But a number of points can be clearly stated. First of all, the apnoea or unequivocally inadequate respiration of the prematurely born infant that nevertheless has a chance of surviving, which is a clinical indication. From a more practical point of view, there is the indication based on the respiratory work: if this is great, as seen in cases of poorly aerated or completely unexpanded lungs; if exhaustion seems imminent; if the child becomes hypoglycaemic due to the laborious respiration and if it becomes metabolically acidotic due to both; and if a severe hypoxia fails to respond to the usual conservative therapy. Under all these conditions, ventilation must be started immediately.

Van der Harten: Was a postmortem performed on the 3 year old child you reported? If so, what were the macroscopic and microscopical findings in the lungs?

Van Zanten: A postmortem was not performed. The only thing I can say is that during the three years over which we followed the child the lungs were radiologically normal, there was no infection of the respiratory tract, and the blood gas values were completely normal, pointing to a normal ventilation-to-perfusion ratio, but these are clinical data.

Van der Harten: Are the lungs of children that survive normal? When they are older as well?

Van Zanten: We should probably say that the length of time for which we have done this work is too short to represent a true follow-up. In fact, this holds for all except a few of our cases.

Polman: For the surviving prematures, what is the situation with respect to the brain and retrolental fibroplasia?

Van Zanten: With respect to the cerebral condition, the answer to the preceding question again holds. This evaluation requires a follow-up lasting for years. It is therefore unknown. Professor van Gelderen has already said that even if children with brain damage have survived, the damage cannot be definitely attributed to the treatment, but that perhaps the positive aspect is that children survive without damage that might have survived damaged if they had been treated conservatively. As far as the retrolental fibroplasia is concerned, it is dependent on the pO_2 in the blood and not on the amount of oxygen supplied to the respiratory tract and lungs. Since we are quite happy if we can achieve a minimally acceptable pO_2 in infants with lung anomalies, the problem of retrolental fibroplasia has actually never come up.

Polman: For a ventilated infant, at what intervals should biochemical checks of pH, pCO_2, calcium, glucose, etc., be performed?

Van Zanten: For calcium and glucose the answer has already been given and lies more in the field of the pediatrician. For the blood gas analysis, on which I should like to give an opinion, it depends on the value reached. As soon as a steady state has been achieved, once a day is usually sufficient and sometimes even once in two days. In the first few hours after ventilation has been instituted, when the lung expansion has perhaps been improved by the ventilation, a blood gas analysis should be done about 15 to 30 minutes after the start of ventilation. If necessary, this is followed by a correction of the ventilation adjustment, with a second check after about two hours, and perhaps another check one or two hours later if an acceptable value has not yet been reached.

Broer: Is there a causal relationship between neonatal shock and on the one hand the hypoperfusion of the lung and on the other inadequate lung expansion, and can you give us additional relevant information on these points?

Van Zanten: It is assumed that there is a causal relationship. On the one hand, the filling of the capillaries of the alveoli gives a certain solidity to the alveolar framework and on the other hand the perfusion of these regions in itself benefits the alveolar cells, often enhancing their capacity to produce a surfactant. Concerning neonatal shock, I can add the following. Many of the infants we have been asked to ventilate had a clinical appearance associated with a state of shock but which did not immediately impress us as such. We administered bicarbonate and some albumin, and we started to ventilate and oxygenate, and these infants improved. But once our attention had been drawn by the literature to the picture of neonatal shock and hypoperfusion of the lung, we went into this point, and I shall cite one example here. This concerns an infant with on almost normal aeration of the lungs but showing the picture of shock. Because cardiac malformations were suspected, a heart catheterization was performed. No cardiac defects were found, but the catheterization did yield some surprising information. Under oxygen administration, the oxygen saturation in the superior caval vein was 3 percent, in the pulmonary artery it was 19 percent, and in the pulmonary vein 86 percent, thus indicating partially unexpanded lungs. In the left ventricle the value was 79 percent, indicating a right-to-left shunt via the foramen ovale; in the descending aorta it was 24 percent, indicating a right-to-left shunt via the ductus Botalli. The blood pressure was the same in the aorta and pulmonary artery (60/45 mm Hg); i.e. low for the aorta and high for the pulmonary artery. We interpreted this picture as a hypocirculation, possibly a hypovolaemia, neonatal shock, resulting in inadequate pulmonary circulation, in turn leading to inadequate tissue perfusion in other parts of the body and giving rise to a metabolic acidosis. Furthermore, the pulmonary anomalies, i.e. the hypoperfusion, and the shunts were responsible for a severe anoxia, again resulting in metabolic acidosis, and the acidosis in turn enhanced the pulmonary vasoconstriction and resistance, which meant that the right-to-left shunt via the ductus Botalli persisted. We supplemented the circulation of this infant by administering 20 percent albumin and we corrected the acidosis, which was severe (pH 6.89 at a pCO_2 of 50). We had to ventilate the infant because of the defective oxygenation. Very slowly, this infant improved. For a long time we continued to find differences in saturation between the heel and the hand, indicating that the ductus Botalli still permitted a right-to-left shunt. But at a certain moment these values became equal and ventilation could be terminated; the infant was discharged in normal health.

Professor Lauweryns then took the floor to answer questions.

De Bruijne: Is it possible that surfactant is destroyed if the alveolar epithelial cells are injured (epithelial necrosis) as a result of the hypoperfusion, and is recovery possible within four or five days?

Lauweryns: The surfactant hypothesis is not a question of true or false. In all probability the surfactant is a substance that is present in varying amounts; it may be absent i.e. in immature fetuses, but I guess it may as well be inhibited, degraded or reappear during the course of a disease (i.e. hyaline membrane disease).

During my lecture I really wanted only to focus the attention on the fact that – in contradistinction to the classic data – we have recently observed typical lamellar bodies and multivesicular bodies in the cylindrical cells of the terminal air buds of an immature baby of 20 weeks' gestational age (240 g.). This could help to explain the findings of Gruenwald who observed by his method good stability of aeration in 40 percent of such fetuses; other authors using the Wilhelmy balance method have not recorded pulmonary surface activity in this group.

Probably the reverse is also true, and much work will have to be done to quantitate the surfactant in the normal fetus and newborn and in various neonatal disorders, and especially the 'idiopathic respiratory distress syndrome' (1, 2).

1. Lauweryns, J., Hyaline membrane disease in newborn infants. Macroscopic, radiographic and light and electron microscopic studies. *Human Pathology* 1, 175–204 (1970).
2. Lauweryns J. and N. Bourgeois, Neonatal hyaline membrane disease: light and electron microscopic studies. Proceedings of the 11th Aspen Emphysema Conference, Aspen, Col. Ed., R. S. Mitchell. *Public Health Service Publication* No. 1879, 3–32. U.S. Government Printing Office, Washington D.C. 1969.

De Bruijne: In most cases for newborn infants we think more of a destruction of surfactant than of its absence.

Lauweryns: This is indeed commonly accepted, but we do not know to what extent it is present nor how much is destroyed; the basic sciences have not yet given us a clue for it. Indeed, the actual surfactant 'measurements' as done on lung extracts i.e. with a Wilhelmy-Langmuir balance, inform us mainly about the presence or the absence of the surfactant in a given patient and allow comparative investigations on a group of patients. But as has been repeatedly pointed out by the specialists in the field, the surfactant balance measurements do not permit to draw quantitative conclusions about the amount of surfactant present.

Koop: Is it possible that the hyaline membranes become more difficult to recognize as such when the neonate is more than a few hours old (for instance, two days)?

Lauweryns: The problem is not that they are more difficult to recognize microscopically. But and as we have shown, the morphologic appearance of the lungs in hyaline membrane disease varies markedly according to the duration of the illness itself after birth and is also influenced by the treatment applied, as discussed by Dr. Gaillard.

Barents: Barcroft has demonstrated intra-uterine respiration in the sheep. What is the divergence from the lung picture you have described as secondary atelectasis? Without mecomium, is this really pathogenetic?

Lauweryns: Your question raises many problems. First, Barcroft (and Vesalius even before him) has indeed demonstrated intra-uterine respiration in the sheep. These early experiments must however be interpreted critically – as has been shown in the more recent literature –, because intra-uterine respiratory movements are stimulated by fetal hypoxemia which has probably not been avoided during these early experiments. We have now indeed available the findings of Adams and his group who have revealed that the up-and-down movement of the amniotic fluid in the fetal lamb probably does not even reach further than the larynx and that aspiration of amniotic fluid in the lungs occurs as a result of an even slight hypoxia.

Secondly, which is the difference between 'the intra-uterine expansion of the lungs with amniotic fluid' and the neonatal 'secondary atelectasis' of which I have shown you examples. I believe it has been Edith Potter who first focused the attention on these various pulmonary expansion types on tissue sections. Due to intra-uterine anoxia or hypoxia, there occurs an aspiration of amniotic fluid in the lungs resulting in a homogeneous and diffuse expansion of all parts of the crumpled, atelectatic fetal lung. In secondary neonatal atelectasis which occurs after birth mostly in premature infants, we observe – as in hyaline membrane disease – a different pulmonary expansion type and picture as I have also shown you, i.e. an irregular air distribution with distended and globulous, perhaps overinflated lobular areas, which alternate with other areas of impressive atelectasis.

The overinflated areas may be lined by hyaline membranes. This pulmonary expansion pattern is best explained by an unequal air distribution due to the absent or diminished occurrence of surfactant. The surfactant is indeed not only an 'anti-atelectatic' or an 'anti-emphysematous' factor, but is also responsible for the pulmonary 'stability' resulting as such in an even and homogeneous air distribution throughout the lung parenchyma.

Ruys: I would like to introduce to you Professor Rosan from the Stanford University. Dr. Gaillard mentioned already his work. He is working now at Leuven at the department of Professor Lauweryns and he will tell us something about his remarkable work.

Rosan: I am surprised and grateful and embarrassed, embarrassed because I cannot talk your language but you can talk mine, embarrassed because I have no tie and embarrassed because my wife waits for me now at the railway station in Amsterdam. It is difficult to summarize six years of work in five minutes. Essentially Dr. Gaillard finds precisely the things

we have found and has added some very important information that we
had suspected, but been unable to get. And this is, that oxygen toxicity is
a function of the prematurity of the infant; the more premature the infant, the less well he will adapt to high concentrations of oxygen. That
is something we have suspected from our animal data and from our human
data but we never really had good data.

I think, I would like to make just one point. There is a pathology treatment, there is a pathology to every treatment.

Once a philosopher said: you cannot observe a thing without changing
it. In medicine we cannot treat a patient without changing him. It is impossible to do that. Anything that we do to the very small premature
infant interferes with some of his adaptive mechanisms. To me the situation is very much as in treatment of cancer of the cervix of the adult. If
you have a woman, who has a stage III cancer you offer her radiation in
the hope that you will cure; you know that some will die; you know that
some will survive and you know that they will be damaged and in some
the damage will be important and in others less and the damage will be
due to the treatment.

You have a desperate disease, you are offering a desperate therapy.
And so it is with the newborn. He has a desperate disease, you offer a
desperate therapy, and there is therefore going to be, there must be,
there will be pathology. It remains to the pathologist to interpret this
damage, to tell you whether or not it is important and to determine what
the course of the damage is on the disease for which the treatment is
offered.

In terms of oxygen, I think our animal work and our human work has
illustrated that on a tissue level the most important kinds of damage that
we can look for, long term chronic damage, assuming that the infant will
survive, are lobular emphysema, which the infant gets because we have
irritated his bronchiole, just like some of you will get it because you
smoke. The infant gets it, the rat gets it, the mouse gets it, the newborn
mouse gets it. And pulmonary hypertension, which the infant gets and at
least morphologically the rat and the mouse and the guinea pig, newborn
mouse and newborn guinea pig. And since the newborn guinea pig is
born in a much different state than the newborn mouse, I think in this
case we can say that the influence of the oxygen must be independent of
the immaturity of the animal. So I think we have to be very careful now as
these children grow and particulary as children who are exposed to
minimal concentrations grow. I think, we have to be very careful of the

bubble-lung syndrome, and the pulmonary hypertension and of documenting carefully what happens to each infant as he is born and as he progresses through life. And I think in that way, you, in your country, with your remarkable high standards of medical care, with your homogeneous population and your ability to follow the patient through his life, I think have a most glorious opportunity to contribute something to an important chapter in pediatric literature, more so I think than any other country in the world. And than the last thing I would like to say is, there are now means by which these diseases can be followed in life and that will involve the pathologist. The pathologist can be brought to a nursery. We have had some experience doing electrophoresis on the secretions of infants who are receiving this treatment, we have done some DNA analysis on the secretions and some were astounding: we had one infant to put out one gram of protein in his endotracheal secretions for every thousand grams of infant over the course of days. We had the opportunity to do exfoliative cytology, which is another way of following the changes in these infants, while they are alive. So I think, although it is true that this is an interdisciplinary meeting and we have much to learn from each other, I think, one of the things perhaps we might keep in mind, is not how we are helping each other but how we can help each other more in the future. Thank you.

Ruys: Professor Rosan, thank you very much for your stimulating and wise words.

Gaillard: I should like to say something concerning the question Professor de Bruijne put to Professor Lauweryns, about whether the cells producing surfactant are destroyed or do not possess the surfactant. In my opinion this is a very fundamental question. And this question is very clearly raised again by Professor Lauweryns's finding that in a small immature fetus we may indeed find the cellular inclusions we previously thought to be the precursor stages of this surfactant. Perhaps it occurs more often; this was of course only an incidental finding. In addition to these two things, i.e. your question and this finding, I should like to mention a finding made by Professor Emery, an English specialist in pediatric pathology, who has made a study in fatal cases of hyaline membrane disease of the costochondral junction and in particular of the enchondral ossification in these regions. Furthermore, Professor Evemark has studied tooth development, in other words regions showing rapid development in this phase. It was found that newborn infants that had succumbed to a hyaline membrane disease invariably showed marked disturbances of the enchondral ossification. And these disturbances can be very clearly followed. You can as it were see from the bit of pathological bone, taking into account the growth rate of this bone, how long ago the disturbances took place. Professor Emery came to the surprising conclusion that this disturbance must have taken place in the intra-uterine period.

The question is, what have enchondral ossification disturbances to do with the hyaline membrane disease? We do not know exactly, but it is conceivable there is a general underlying, rather chronic disorder that can lead to a disturbance in regions of high cellular activity and perhaps also in the cells responsible for the production of surfactant. This is of course only a hypothesis requiring proof or disproof, but it in any case has the usefulness of drawing etiological speculation back to the intra-uterine period.

INDEX OF SUBJECTS